CENTER FOR APPLIED RESEARCH, INC.
3600 MARKET STREET
SUITE 501
PHILADELPHIA, PA. 19104

# The Physician-Manager Alliance

Stephen M. Davidson
Marion McCollom
Janelle Heineke

# The
# Physician-Manager Alliance

. . . . . . . . . . . . . . . . . . . . . . . . . . . . . .

## Building the Healthy
## Health Care Organization

Jossey-Bass Publishers
San Francisco

. . . . . . . . . . . . . .

Substantial discounts on bulk quantities of Jossey-Bass books are available to corporations, professional associations, and other organizations. For details and discount information, contact the special sales department at Jossey-Bass Inc., Publishers (415) 433–1740; Fax (800) 605–2665.

For sales outside the United States, please contact your local Simon & Schuster International Office.

 Manufactured in the United States of America on Lyons Falls Pathfinder Tradebook. This paper is acid-free and 100 percent totally chlorine-free.

**Library of Congress Cataloging-in-Publication Data**

Davidson, Stephen M.
 The physician-manager alliance : building the healthy health care organization / Stephen M. Davidson, Marion McCollom, Janelle Heineke. — 1st ed.
   p.   cm.
 Includes bibliographical references and index.
 ISBN 0–7879–0215–2
 1. Managed care plans (Medical care)—United States—Administration.  2. Medicine—Practice—United States.  3. Health services administration—United States—Quality control.
 I. McCollom, Marion, date.  II. Heineke, Janelle N.  III. Title.
 [DNLM: 1. Delivery of Health Care—organization & administration—United States.  2. Health Services—organization & administration—United States.  3. Physician's Role.  W 84 AA1 D23p 1996]
RA413.5.U5D38  1996
362.1'0425—dc20                                                          95–43901

*HB Printing*          10  9  8  7  6  5  4  3  2  1                    FIRST EDITION

# Contents

· · · · · · · · · · · · · · · · · · · · · · · · · · · · · · · ·

# Preface

Everyone has a stake in how well the health care system performs. All of us—even those who today are the youngest and healthiest among us—are likely someday to need care for a serious illness or injury. Those with other relationships to the health care system— such as clinical professionals who deliver the services we all may use, or managers of the organizations under whose auspices that care is delivered—have additional reasons to be interested in its performance.

However many connections we have, and whatever their level of intensity, all of us have a common interest in the way the care-giving aspect of the health care system is adapting to the dramatic changes of the last twenty years or more. Can we still count on physicians to focus primarily on our needs as patients, or do some of the new financial arrangements create competing priorities for them? Have the health care organizations on which so many of us depend mastered the complexities of delivering the benefits of modern medicine? Can we have confidence that needed referrals will be made smoothly and in a timely fashion without harm to us? Does the fact that more clinicians work for or under the auspices of health care organizations make the competent delivery of complicated services more certain, or do loyalties to the organization intrude on their first commitment to patients? Are the stories of errors and horrors that appear daily in newspapers—accidental overdoses of powerful drugs, amputation of the wrong leg—just isolated incidents in a system that is basically sound? Or are they the tip of an iceberg, hiding common instances of carelessness and poor judgment that escape our attention because the patient recovered?

We have written this book because, first, whatever the answers, it is only prudent to take the reasonableness of these questions as a warning. Two recent books reveal the risks in very human terms. In one (Gilbert, 1995), the widow of an English professor wrote about her husband's avoidable death following surgery for prostate cancer. The surgery was relatively common and the risk of internal bleeding was well known, but test results revealing signs of massive hemorrhaging were missed until it was too late to save him. Although the surgeon was a distinguished physician, the other staff were experienced, and the hospital had a good reputation, the patient died prematurely because they failed to exercise reasonable care.

In the second book (Heymann, 1995), a young physician recounted not only her own story as a patient with a serious and unexpected illness but also those of other patients. In many instances, physicians and other clinical staff simply ignored complaints and questions from patients that could have saved enormous amounts of suffering, not to mention money, and in some cases, lives. Some of those patients were themselves physicians, who could articulate what was happening to them in the language of the professionals who were caring for them. The fact that even they could not get their caregivers to take seriously their complaints of symptoms or pain makes it easy to understand why the rest of us, when we become patients, have trouble being heard. More important than that, however, the cumulative effect of the tales she recounts seriously undermines our confidence in the health care system as a whole. Above all, patients must be able to expect that when they put themselves in the hands of a professional, the benefits they receive will be limited only by the nature of their medical condition and the state of medical knowledge about it.

We are concerned that the complexity of much modern medical care increases the risks from acute illness. An episode often has many segments, and even though each part should be connected smoothly to the next, many patients get lost in the transitions from one professional to another. (See, for example, the story "Uncoordinated Care" in Chapter Six.) In addition, the organizations in which many clinical professionals work are themselves sometimes barriers to good care because among other things they may inadvertently dilute the individual professional's sense of responsibility for his or her patient.

The second reason we have written this book is as important as the first: we believe good management can create conditions that greatly reduce the risks of poor care. Indeed, the stakes represented by the lives and health of individuals *demand* that obstacles to good care be identified and removed. But while the risks will increase as the role of organizations in the delivery of services continues to grow, the opportunities to shrink those risks will also improve. For one thing, the best chance to integrate seamlessly the disparate elements of complicated episodes of care may be when all the participants are part of a single organization. In addition, only organizations have the capital to obtain the expensive machines, including linked computers, that can benefit patients during episodes of illness. Third, a relatively new entity, the managed care organization, has advantages that at least in theory should permit it to conserve limited resources by delivering even ambulatory services more efficiently than the decentralized, fragmented system most of us grew up with.

What will it take for hospitals, managed care organizations, and others to reach their potential, and by doing so restore confidence in the health care system? We believe the answer is for managers, who have primary responsibility for the organizations from which most Americans now obtain their care, and the doctors, who have primary responsibility for providing that care, to engage one another in deliberate efforts to achieve that critical goal. Together they must develop policies and procedures that increase the probability that patient encounters with the health care system will produce the hoped-for health status improvements and decrease the probability of avoidable error. It is no longer enough to rely on the skill and commitment of individual clinicians; the system has become so complex that too much is beyond their control. Nor is it enough to assume that the mere creation of entities with such names as physician-hospital organizations (PHOs) or integrated delivery systems (IDSs) or integrated service networks (ISNs) means either that physicians and managers are working well together or that integration in the delivery of services has actually occurred and the complexity of the caregiving process has been tamed.

Moreover, the efforts of even the most dedicated managers and physicians to find better ways to deliver care will be made much more difficult by the constraints under which medicine is practiced in the contemporary United States: the relentless preoccupation with the cost of care, increasingly competitive health care markets, and a large and growing minority of Americans who have no health insurance coverage. In such an environment, many physicians work under incentives, pressures, and constraints that may compete with their obligation to their patients.

The pace of change in the U.S. health care system has not been slowed by the failure of efforts in Washington and in many state capitals to enact reform legislation. Yet, we believe that the implications of the changes that are occurring—especially for the delivery of effective medical services—are not fully understood, that some of them create challenges that have not been fully recognized to date, and that the continued failure to confront and overcome those challenges is harmful to the health of all of us. Understanding the risks inherent in the turbulence of our health care system is a necessary first step toward effective action to reduce them.

## Audience

This book is addressed primarily to the managers and doctors who must work together to make the care we depend upon reliable enough to inspire confidence. It is made necessary by three of the most important changes that have occurred in the health care system: (1) the growth of organizations as the source of not only our insurance but also our health care services, (2) the fierce competitiveness of a growing number of markets, and (3) the increasing complexity of much medical care.

As a result of the first change, organizations have become much more important, and their role in the delivery of services has changed in critical ways. Hospitals are no longer just "the doctors' workshop." Most Americans now have access to a physician primarily through managed care organizations, which are paid in ways that give them an interest in limiting expenditures on services, if not the services themselves. The second large change, increasing price competition in health care markets, creates conflicting imperatives for insurers and managed care organizations. At the same time that it pressures them to *expand their offerings* in order to be more attractive than other organizations in the feverish effort to attract subscribers, it also leads them to *restrict the care* actually provided in order to control expenditures on care and keep their premium prices low. For reasons we discuss in the book, many of the decisions they have made place arbitrary limits on services to which patients are entitled—limits based not on individual need but on the organization's policy—or create hurdles physicians must jump in order to do what their medical judgment tells them is best for their patients. Third, medical care has become more complex, often requiring links between professionals and sometimes between organizations. Linkages take time, which costs money, but clinicians are under pressure to be "productive" and to keep costs down.

These developments have changed the context of medical care so much that no one—not physicians, managers, patients, or payers—is content with the relationships that are evolving. Comfortable new patterns of behavior have not yet developed, and constructive new relationships between doctors and managers have not yet emerged in most health care organizations. We are in a transition period between the medical care system that evolved slowly and incrementally from the late nineteenth century through the mid 1960s, giving everyone a chance to experiment until they found the best ways to adapt, and the current scene in which the pace of innovation has been so fast that participants have had difficulty adjusting and creating a new equilibrium.

## Purpose of the Book

This book focuses on the delivery of services in health care organizations. One goal is to provide a context that makes clear not only the risks of failing to learn how to provide good services in organizations, but also the opportunities in effectively linking management processes and caregiving. While some have argued that the successful use of the methods of continuous quality improvement (CQI) or total quality management (TQM) in other enterprises could be emulated in the health care system, too many key players in the health care drama still ignore the fundamental precepts of these tools (Blumenthal & Scheck, 1995). To cover their failure to adopt these methods, some have used rhetoric that makes it appear that they are implementing them. But there is still too much resistance from managers who do not want to share power with physicians and from doctors who often denigrate managers as mere bureaucrats. Many managers consider doctors unwilling to face the "realities" of the modern health care system, while many doctors argue that managers are more concerned about market share and the bottom line than about service to patients or about quality of care. In such an electric atmosphere, the rhetoric is charged, and progress is slow and painful.

We believe that the conditions that made it possible for this kind of antagonism to be tolerated without seriously undermining patient care have changed and continue to change in ways that dramatically increase the stakes for all of us. In this book, instead of describing methods of CQI or TQM, we begin a step further back in the logic chain. We argue not only that serious attention must be given to organization-based care as a phenomenon but also that the only way for health care organizations to achieve their mission in modern society is for managers and doctors to work together. It will not be sufficient for managers to impose productivity "standards" of so many patient visits per hour or per day or to require that physicians get permission from nurse-reviewers before providing certain services. Managers must create internal systems that help physicians take better care of patients, and doctors must help managers keep the organizations functioning effectively and efficiently.

Finally, although we argue that a *partnership* between managers and physicians is crucial to a successful future, we put the primary burden on managers to create the conditions that make such a partnership possible and to take the initiative to engage physicians in the process of building that collaboration. But where managers fail to act, doctors need to step in to enlist managers in building the necessary collaboration.

## Overview of the Contents

In Chapter One we introduce the main themes of the book: that organizations have become the *mainstream* of American medicine and that this trend creates new challenges for the health care field. We illustrate the nature and variety of challenges in our organization-based health care system with a series of vignettes designed to put a human face to these abstractions.

In Chapter Two we provide data to demonstrate that organizations have come to dominate the health care field. In Chapters Three and Four we discuss the evolving health care system from two perspectives: first, that of purchasers, including ordinary citizens and the employers who pay for much of the private coverage we depend on; then that of providers, especially the doctors and managers whose roles in the new health care system are both critical and continually changing.

Chapter Five presents a picture of health care delivered according to the standard that we as a society need to demand from our health care system. The chapter describes what we call "the healthy health care organization," one from which people receive care that is responsive to their needs, timely, considerate, and technologically appropriate. Moreover, in such an organization, the several elements of care—including referrals and procedures performed away from the site of the original encounter—are seamlessly integrated with one another.

Having described care the way it *ought* to be, we turn in Chapter Six to describe care the way it really tends to be practiced in organizations. We present two case examples that illustrate many of the problems that arise in a health care system that is capable of great achievements when care is delivered through organizations. We identify the challenges facing the two key groups of actors, doctors and managers, as well as some of the obstacles they must overcome and some of the tools with which they have to work.

In preparation for providing practical guidance to managers and doctors, we take a step back in Chapter Seven, to summarize several theoretical perspectives on physician-manager relationships. Out of a conviction that people can solve problems best when they understand *why* a phenomenon occurs and *why* they should take steps to correct it, we consider this discussion of theory to be quite practical.

In Chapter Eight we synthesize some of the lessons from the perspectives discussed in Chapter Seven to present what we think of as an eclectic approach to improving the delivery of health care through organizations. We illustrate this conviction by showing how it aids better understanding of some of the stories we presented in Chapter One as illustrations of problems.

Finally, in Chapter Nine we present some practical suggestions for managers about how to approach the challenges they face. Since each situation is unique and each solution must be tailored to those special conditions, this is not a "cookbook," but rather a general approach or orientation that can be applied to many situations.

The book is organized as a progression of steps: from recognition of a set of problems, to articulation of a goal, to a diagnosis of the

causes of dysfunctions, and finally to suggestions based on the understanding that results when those theoretical insights are applied to
the practical challenges faced by health care managers. By taking
this approach, our hope is that managers and doctors will be able to
embrace our suggestions with a conviction that comes from having
proceeded along this path with us.

## Acknowledgments

We are pleased to acknowledge our debt to the Robert Wood Johnson Foundation, especially Lewis Sandy and Beth Stevens, who
encouraged us from the beginning and then facilitated our efforts
to transform into this book the report we submitted to the foundation. They and we hope this book will increase the value of the
foundation's investment.

We appreciate the support and encouragement of Deans Louis
Lataif and Edwin Murray as we labored to complete work on the
book. Davidson is particularly appreciative of a year-long sabbati-
cal that freed up enough time to complete the project while it is still
timely. He also gratefully acknowledges the additional support for
this work provided by John Snow, Inc., of Boston, particularly the
encouragement of Joel Lamstein, the firm's president, and Patricia
Fairchild, vice president.

Our research assistants, Ray Blaisdell, Robert Kaplan, and Jen-
nifer Lee, helped in many ways, not all of which were mundane or
tedious.

We owe a special debt of gratitude to the multidisciplinary panel
of experts who read a draft of the report we prepared for the foundation and who spent a stimulating and, for us, very profitable day in
Princeton sharing their insights on the issues the report raised. They
were Harris Berman, CEO of the Tufts Associated Health Plans;
Michael Stuart, then director of medical education at the Group
Health Cooperative of Puget Sound; Kenneth Bloem, then CEO
of Stanford University Hospital; Sister Angela Bontempo, former

hospital chief executive in the Daughters of Charity National Health Care System; W. Richard Scott, Stanford University sociologist; Curtis McLaughlin, professor of operations management, University of North Carolina, Chapel Hill; Martin Charns, director, Management Decision Research Center, Department of Veterans Affairs; and W. Pete Welch, health care economist at the Urban Institute in Washington.

Several physicians and managers read parts or all of the book in draft. Their efforts were beyond the call of duty, and we benefited greatly from their willingness to share their experience: Stephen Schoenbaum, Robert Buxbaum, Daniel Reardon, Mark Robbins, and three anonymous reviewers.

While we are exceedingly grateful for the help provided by all of these knowledgeable people, and we believe the book is better for their generosity, they are not responsible for our failure to correct any errors that remain.

Finally, in a book that extols the virtues of partnership, it is only fitting that we acknowledge the many contributions of our life partners, Harriet, Tom, and George, who helped sustain us throughout the long months of effort that resulted in this book.

*Boston, Massachusetts*  
*November 1995*

Stephen M. Davidson  
Marion McCollom  
Janelle Heineke

# The Authors

. . . . . . . . . . . . . . . . . . . . . . . . . . . . . .

**Stephen M. Davidson** is associate professor of health care management and management policy and former director of the Graduate
Program in Health Care Management (1985–1990) at Boston University School of Management. He is also director of research at
John Snow, Inc., a public health–oriented consulting, training, and
research firm headquartered in Boston. He earned a B.A. degree
(1961) in political science from Swarthmore College and a Ph.D.
degree (1974) from the University of Chicago. He has taught health
policy and management for more than twenty years, first at the University of Chicago and then at Northwestern University's Kellogg
Graduate School of Management before joining the faculty at
Boston University.

Davidson has been an active researcher for many years on a variety of issues related to the organization, financing, and delivery of
health care services. Much of his work has centered on the role of
physicians in the changing health care system. He conducted a
study of factors associated with physician participation in Medicaid
in thirteen states, and a study of utilization and expenditures in a
prepaid managed care experiment in Suffolk County, New York.
More recently, he completed a study of physician retention in community health centers and examined physician participation in a
mandatory managed care initiative in the Maryland Medicaid program (along with collaborators from the Center for Health Affairs at

Project HOPE). Currently, he is working (with James H. Maxwell) on an examination of the behavior of large companies that purchase health insurance for their employees.

He has consulted with a variety of health care organizations, and has authored or coauthored two previous books, *Medicaid Decisions: A Systematic Analysis of the Cost Problem* (1980) and *The Cost of Living Longer: National Health Insurance and the Elderly* (1980); several monographs and book chapters; and numerous articles in leading professional journals, including *Medical Care*, *Journal of Health Politics*, *Policy and Law*, and *Health Affairs*.

**Marion McCollom** has taught organizational behavior since 1986 at Boston University's School of Management, where she is currently associate professor. She teaches in the MBA, doctoral, and undergraduate programs and in 1994 was named faculty director of the MBA program, responsible for launching the school's new MBA curriculum. She has also served on the core faculties of Boston University's Executive MBA and Leadership Institute programs. She received her A.B. degree magna cum laude (1972) from Harvard University, her M.P.P.M. degree (1982) from the Yale University School of Management, and a Ph.D. degree (1987), with distinction, from Yale University.

McCollom consults to a variety of organizations, focusing primarily on improving work relationships and developing effective decision-making processes. She has published numerous scholarly articles on organization culture, organizational narratives, and the structure and dynamics of family-owned business. She coedited *Groups in Context: A New Perspective on Group Dynamics* (1990) and is currently working on another coauthored book, on family business (forthcoming from Harvard Business School Press, with Kelin Gersick, John Davis, and Ivan Lansberg).

**Janelle Heineke** is assistant professor of operations management at Boston University School of Management. She earned a B.S.N.

degree (1975) from Marquette University, an M.S.N. degree (1979) from Boston College, and an M.B.A. degree (1988) from Babson College before completing her D.B.A. degree (1992) at Boston University. She has more than fifteen years of clinical health care experience, practicing as an obstetrics/gynecology nurse practitioner for ten years. She also has ten years of health care industry management experience in hospitals and HMOs.

Heineke currently teaches quality management, service operations management, and general operations management. Her main research interest is the management of technical professionals, especially in service industries. She has conducted research on the effect of management decisions on clinical outcomes in HMOs and has published papers in *Quality Progress, The California Management Review, Operations Management Review,* and *The International Journal of Operations and Production Management.*

# The Physician-Manager Alliance

# The High Stakes of Change
## The Need for Physician-Manager Alliances

This book is about the relationships between doctors and the managers of health care organizations. It grows out of the recognition that these organizations have become increasingly prominent on the U.S. health care scene and that most physicians do increasing amounts of their professional work under organizational auspices. It also derives from our conviction that, given these conditions, managers will attempt to influence the patterns of health care services delivered in or through organizations.

Organizations that sell products or services have a stake in the work of the employees and contractors who produce those products or services; therefore, the managers who are responsible for an organization's viability and who will not want to leave the performance of that work to chance *must* attempt to influence it. In health care organizations, the service being offered is care for patients, and the people who produce it are clinicians. Thus, managers will want to assure themselves that the organization's services are responsive to patients who otherwise would go elsewhere for their care, that the quality is adequate to produce good health, and that the organization does not waste resources and thus jeopardize its viability by spending more to deliver the care than it collects in revenue.

For many, the notion that physicians will be managed is offensive. Doctors, after all, are the caregiving professionals we rely on when we are most vulnerable. Their entire commitment, an essential element of their ancient code of ethics, is to their patients. They cannot be managed, many people will say. In fact, they *should not* be managed. Perhaps *care* can be managed, but if so, it is the doctors who must do it.

Nonetheless, for the reasons indicated, managers *will* attempt to manage doctors. The only questions are, how will they do it? What goals will they be trying to achieve? What effects, both intended and unintended, will they produce?

This book also grows out of a deep concern that as a general rule the management functions related to the delivery of services are neither well understood nor well performed in health care organizations. As evidence, we cite the frequent complaints of physicians that they have lost their autonomy; that they are spending endless amounts of time with paperwork to justify services they "know" are right; that managers, responding to the dominant concern of payers to save money, want physicians to practice "cookbook" medicine; and that clerks who do not understand patients' needs are deciding what services physicians can provide. On the flip side of the complaints are physicians' boasts that they have learned how to answer the questions or fill out the forms so as to get their way with the bureaucrats.

For their part, managers are unhappy, too. Although they feel forced by the payers' preoccupation with costs and the fierce competition of many health care markets to deal with clinicians about clinical matters, most managers would prefer not to have to do so. Since they understand all too well that physicians know more than they do about medicine, managers tend not to discuss medical issues because they know they will be unable to respond to the technical points they expect doctors to raise. Instead, when they do get involved, managers tend to focus on process, emphasizing work rules—how many patients should be seen in an hour, how long the average visit should be—or cost-control measures, such as limiting the list of drugs that doctors can use to treat particular conditions. Having to make clinical decisions in these circumstances only increases the anger of doctors who believe that the rules hamper their ability to serve their patients well. Because rules tend to lump together everyone sharing an important characteristic—a diagnosis, for example—the result is to deny physicians the ability to exercise their professional judgment and make the adjustments they think will result in better care for the individual patient. A physician's judgment may sometimes turn out to be wrong, but after all, patients have other characteristics besides diagnoses, any one of which can render a policy that would be appropriate in most situations less than optimal in a given instance.

Why is this a problem? Managers are just doing their job. They are charged with ensuring the organization's viability; we must assume they are doing what they think is necessary to accomplish that goal. Moreover, doctors can be difficult, too; and those who are unhappy with the way they are treated by managers can escape an organization by resigning. Actually, since so much care is now delivered through organizations, complete avoidance of managers is becoming less and less possible. The physician who wants to continue to practice medicine may find his or her options limited to looking for a *different* health care organization.

Managers who are unhappy at the prospect of having to raise difficult questions with physicians in a situation that puts them at a disadvantage could also, theoretically, avoid the issues. They could hire well-trained, experienced physicians and just assume they are delivering good care. If that does not work, they could avoid unpleasant debates and personal acrimony by writing out policies in memos. Indeed, this practice is fairly common. But, of course, when the written policies are controversial, they too can create hard feelings that sometimes lead to open confrontation.

The fact is, too many managers and doctors prefer to avoid each other, and when they cannot avoid contact, their actions often have the effect, intentionally or not, of widening the gulf between them.

The stakes are too high—for patients, for physicians, and for health care organizations—for these patterns to continue. Managers have the responsibility to create conditions that make it possible for conscientious, well-trained clinicians to deliver good care in a timely, efficient manner. Then, having created those conditions (which they must continue to refine), they must stay informed about physician performance in order to assure themselves that the clinicians are in fact delivering good care. When they are not satisfied with what they find, managers must work with physician colleagues to discover what the impediments to satisfactory results are and remove them. Unless managers succeed at these responsibilities, their organizations may not survive in an increasingly constrained market. Patients will be poorly served, and doctors will be not only unhappy but ineffective as well.

## The Need for Action

Four factors create the imperative for managers to install and refine conditions that permit, encourage, and facilitate the provision of good and efficient care by physicians.

First, care has become much more complex. In a single episode of illness it is common for sick patients to receive services from multiple professionals, often at different locations and in different organizations. Moreover, these services increasingly involve expensive technology. Modern medicine creates a need for smooth handoffs of patients from one professional to another, and for complex information systems that are paradoxically simple to the user yet able to clarify the pattern of care for managers.

The second factor is that the American health care system is becoming more and more constrained financially. In the old days of cost-based reimbursement, it did not seem to matter much if a patient received more tests than the doctor really needed in order to diagnose a condition or assess progress; insurers paid what providers billed. Nor did it matter if an extra set of X-rays were taken because the technician took the first set of the wrong leg or ribs; no one was hurt, and those costs were covered, too. But in fact it did matter. Costs rose steadily, and wasteful habits were formed and reinforced. Now, costs have risen so high that many employers are either cutting back the health insurance benefits they make available to their employees or dropping health care coverage altogether. In addition, the wasteful habits formed in the days of cost-based reimbursement are proving hard to change. Unless such waste is eliminated, many Americans will be unable to benefit from the impressive scientific gains of recent years.

Third, in a highly mobile population many patients find it hard to establish and maintain long-term relationships with primary care physicians. So many Americans move each year—both laypersons and physicians—that even if patients find a physician who is responsive and attentive and in whom they feel confidence, chances are good that within a few short years that tie will be broken.

Finally, and perhaps most important, more and more Americans receive their care through or in organizations, and more and more physicians are employees of health care organizations or have contracts with them to deliver services. To some degree, Americans whose relationships with individual physicians are disrupted look toward organizations to provide a continuing connection with the health care system. Increasingly, *health care organizations are the mainstream* of American medicine. It is not an exaggeration, therefore, to say that *most* Americans will be affected by how well these organizations and their clinicians deliver services.

Fortunately, at the same time that modern medicine is facing these new challenges, certain tools are now available to both managers and physicians that make it possible to improve care *and* increase productivity. Chief among them is the computer, which can store vast quantities of information yet make that information accessible and useful in identifying problems, suggesting solutions, and monitoring progress.

Thus, we are at a point when managers have responsibility for much health care and its effects even though they are not clinicians. Since they do not deliver the services themselves, managers *must* deal with physicians. For their part, physicians *must* do things they did not need to do before:

- Physicians must be concerned about transferring patients and patient information to other clinicians in "handoffs" that, if they occurred at all in the past, tended to be much simpler.

- They must be concerned about costs, which in the past they frequently did not know about and certainly did not worry about.

- They must continue to keep up with the explosion of information regarding new treatments and services and, sometimes, new diseases.

- Whereas in the past, hospital-based physicians expected managers simply to make the physical plant and financial systems operate smoothly, now they must rely on managers for information and the other resources—including patients—that make it possible for them to practice modern medicine.

Thus, physicians *depend* on managers, but they also mistrust or even fear them, because managers also monitor the care physicians provide and the expenditures incurred in providing it. Although past interactions and relationships of physicians and managers may not have been particularly pleasant, it is no longer acceptable that they cope with their mutual discomfort by *avoiding* serious engagement with one another. Since both have critical, though different, roles to play in the delivery of services, they must find ways to work together.

In the effort to achieve this difficult objective, we put the primary burden on the managers, in hospitals, health maintenance organizations (HMOs), preferred provider organizations (PPOs), and physician-hospital organizations (PHOs), among others. Managers must not only create conditions that enable physicians to perform at their best, but they must also hold physicians accountable for meeting the high standards of their profession. Having said this, however, we do not mean to suggest that managers must be dominant over physicians, or that physicians have no obligation to make the system work better. Instead, we believe it is the managers' responsibility to develop and nurture the organizational environment that makes possible the working partnership we believe is necessary today. The health care organization is their responsibility, and making it work is their charge.

Thus managers' interest in clinical care is both legitimate and essential to achieving quality health care that will satisfy everyone, including the clinicians who provide it and the patients who seek and use it. At the same time that we recognize the legitimacy and importance of managers' interest in clinical matters, we also believe that physicians must have clinical autonomy in their decision making with individual patients. When considering what tests to order and what treatment to use with a particular patient, the physician must be free to use his or her best clinical judgment. He or she must not be constrained by arbitrary rules that place each patient into a category and define appropriate treatment according to the characteristics common to that group. Only if the physician has the freedom to make clinical decisions will patients have confidence that they have received the services most likely to help them, and only in this way will physicians believe they have followed the high standards of their profession. Conversely, even when they are free of interference in specific clinical decisions, physicians often make those decisions ignorant of the costs of alternative treatments. Either managers have not calculated those costs (cost accounting in health care is difficult and state-of-the-art accounting practices are still not pervasive in the field) or they know the costs but have not communicated them to the clinicians.

While at first glance these two principles—managerial involvement and physician autonomy—may appear to be contradictory, we believe not only that they are compatible but also that they must coexist. *The professional challenge for managers and physicians alike is therefore to discover ways to live by both principles simultaneously.*

We do not ask you, the reader, to accept this position at face value. Indeed, an important purpose of the book is to persuade you of its validity. To begin that effort, we present some brief vignettes to demonstrate (1) that the delivery of services in or through health care organizations creates serious problems; (2) that these problems are felt by all groups who have contact with the health care system—patients, physicians, and managers; and (3) that the problems occur at any point at which individuals interact with a health care organization—from the patient's initial effort to purchase coverage, through the first contact in an illness episode, at any point during its course, and even afterwards, when the issue may simply be paying a bill. These vignettes (which play out primarily in the context of patients' attempts to seek care and physicians' efforts to provide it) are not intended to assign blame for the problems to any one group. Indeed, since managers, physicians, and patients alike share culpability for the breakdowns we describe, each must play a role in solving them. We believe strongly, however, that in this effort it is managers who must create the environment and set the tone for delivery of good service by physicians, who are the organization's principal contact with patients.

Throughout the book we offer other illustrative examples. All are true. Those taken from published sources are identified as such. In some cases, the text is verbatim from the original source; in others, the original is paraphrased and shortened. Those not identified as being from a published document were obtained by the authors in interviews. In such cases, personal characteristics of the subjects, including names, are disguised to protect their privacy, but the facts are as we learned them.

## Evidence of Problems: The Patient's View

As more and more Americans are being encouraged or even forced by their employers to subscribe to managed care organizations

(MCOs), patient concerns about where the loyalties of the organizations lie are of more than academic interest.

Here is an account of the efforts of one person to be a rational consumer.

* * * * * * *

## Enrolling in an HMO

Sarah Redfield (a pseudonym), the former general counsel for a major New York teaching hospital, contracted breast cancer and explored the possibility of joining an HMO. She called six major HMOs operating in New York, saying she was looking for one to join and asking for information. She said the first problem was simply finding the right person to talk to. Multiple calls were necessary at each plan, and at one, she never found anyone knowledgeable enough to answer her questions.

In choosing an HMO, a central question is which doctors provide services under its aegis, but only two of the six that Sarah investigated would identify the plan's cancer specialists for her. Moreover, while a key element of HMO operations is that the patient's primary care physician provides access to specialists by making referrals, several plans required that the primary care physician also approve the specific treatments the specialist ordered.

Only four of the six plans would send her a copy of the contract that spelled out the terms of membership, and to get three of them, she had to persist with multiple calls. Moreover, three plans required a check for the first premium with the application form even though the typical applicant would not yet, if ever, have seen the contract.

One of the reasons the contract is important is that although all the plans distribute summaries of their services, only three sent lists of exclusions. Moreover, according to this HMO shopper, many of the exclusions were quite general, and it was difficult to figure out when they would apply. Sarah noted that even services that would seem to be covered must be approved at the time they are needed. And because approvals are given on a case-by-case basis, a patient cannot really know what coverage is available before selecting a plan. Sarah quoted one plan's representative as saying, "You don't know until you actually hand in that claim form."

The woman summarized her saga in these terms: "If I had trouble getting information from the HMOs, I can only imagine what it must be like for other people—those who aren't lawyers with health care expertise" (Rosenfeld, 1994, p. A23).

♦ ♦ ♦ ♦ ♦ ♦ ♦

If health care organizations will not even provide accurate and complete information to a prospective customer, then clearly service to a clientele is not their primary orientation. Moreover, it does not matter whether the breakdown in this particular case represented a deliberate effort to discourage a potential high-use patient from subscribing or was merely inadvertent. In the first instance, the organization would have been guilty of protecting itself from the high costs associated with the treatment of cancer; in the latter, of sloppiness, demonstrating poor quality control (here, of the marketing function).

It is not only in the "business" functions that problems exist. As the next vignette shows, they can also be found in the delivery of services, where for patients who have cleared the enrollment hurdle the stakes can be much higher.

♦ ♦ ♦ ♦ ♦ ♦ ♦

### Waiting to Be Seen

Dave Michaels, a healthy, middle-class man, was riding his bicycle for exercise and was hit by a car; the driver had been distracted and did not see the bike rider approaching the intersection from the right. Dave was knocked off his bike and his head hit the ground. Although he was wearing a helmet, he

suffered a severe headache and possible concussion. A passerby
stopped, checked on Dave's condition, and drove him to the
nearby office of his staff-model HMO. There, Dave went to the
desk of the particular practice group in which he was enrolled,
explained the situation, asked to be seen, and took a seat in the
waiting room. Some time later, he asked the receptionist for
some aspirin for his headache. He spent part of the next several
hours lying on the carpeted floor of the waiting room because he
was too dizzy and nauseated to sit in a chair. It was not until
four hours after arriving at the center that he was finally able to
see a physician. While he waited, no one performed a triage
examination or even checked his blood pressure.

◆ ◆ ◆ ◆ ◆ ◆ ◆

As it turned out, Dave had not suffered a concussion and the
delay had caused him no real physical harm. It is also true, however,
that the nurse-receptionist made no effort either to expedite his
being seen by one of the several physicians in the practice or to
respond to his obvious discomfort. Although his care was clearly
inadequate, this patient was not feeling strong enough to be a force-
ful advocate for his own treatment. The HMO may not have had
standard procedures for staff in the practices to determine and meet
an injured patient's needs, or it may have had such procedures but
had inadequate supervision to ensure that such a patient would be
treated appropriately. Regardless, the particular nurse-receptionist
on duty did not take the initiative to determine the patient's need
and see that it was met in a timely manner. If the patient had been
accompanied by a friend or relative who was able to insist on his
being seen, perhaps staff would have responded more appropriately.
But an organization must establish and meet its own standards of
good quality.

A key element in managed care is the patient's association with
a single primary care physician. On the most superficial level, this
formal connection is intended to provide some order and continu-
ity to the individual's use of services. A patient has access to the

organization's range of services only through the primary care physician, who not only furnishes first-contact care during an episode of illness but is also expected to guide the patient's use of ancillary, specialty, and hospital services as well. On another level, these rules provide an opportunity for the two people to build a relationship that can help reduce the impersonality of a large organization. In addition, as we argue later, good doctor-patient relationships can contribute to both greater efficiency and better patient compliance with the physician's recommendations, resulting in a more secure quality of services. The next two examples report patient experiences with their primary care physicians.

♦ ♦ ♦ ♦ ♦ ♦ ♦

## The Patient's Personal Physician

Ann Green, a high-school junior playing third base on the girls' varsity softball team, was knocked over by an opposing base runner barrelling into third base. As she tried to pick herself up off the ground after the play, she discovered she could not stand because of a severe pain in the area of her left knee. Her mother, who was a spectator at the game, called her physician's office at the staff-model HMO to which they belonged and was instructed to bring Ann in. They arrived shortly thereafter, at about 4:45 P.M.., and were told by the receptionist that Ann's primary care physician, Dr. Lee, was with a patient and was scheduled to leave at five. She promised to tell Dr. Lee that Ann was there and reassured her that Ann would be seen shortly.

At 5:10, after several inquiries about when Ann, who was becoming increasingly uncomfortable, could be seen, Mrs. Green was told that Dr. Lee had left for the evening and that Dr. Stone, another physician in the practice, would see Ann. They were ushered into an examining room where Dr. Stone examined Ann, determined that no bones were broken, provided some medication to relieve the pain, and wrote out a referral to an orthopedist. Mrs. Green was advised to call the orthopedic clinic in the morning to arrange an appointment for Ann to be seen.

◆ ◆ ◆ ◆ ◆ ◆ ◆

From the standpoint of measurable medical outcomes, Ann Green received appropriate care: she was told to come to the medical center, was seen by a physician within half an hour, and was referred to the appropriate specialist. The critical fact that Ann had chosen Dr. Lee as her primary care physician turned out to be irrelevant to Dr. Lee. When five o'clock came and her scheduled workday ended, the doctor left the building; by her action, she communicated to her patient that she did not value the doctor-patient relationship. Moreover, she left by a back door, thus avoiding the waiting room where Ann and her mother (who was also a patient of Dr. Lee's) were sitting. She left without taking a couple of minutes to ask Ann, whom she had seen several times for routine matters, how she was feeling and to reassure her that even though Dr. Lee had to leave, Ann would be in good hands with Dr. Stone. As we note later, quality-of-care theorists consider that the affective side of patient-physician encounters, which influences patient satisfaction and confidence, contributes to overall quality of care and to patients' perceptions of the outcomes of care.

◆ ◆ ◆ ◆ ◆ ◆ ◆

### Failing to Communicate

Marilyn Edwards, a woman in her late thirties and in generally good health, had been a member of an HMO for almost ten years. She had been seeing Dr. Simon for about five years. Marilyn's prior physician, with whom she had established what she considered to be a good professional relationship, had recommended Dr. Simon as her replacement when she left the practice to move to another state.

Marilyn called the plan to make an appointment with Dr. Simon because of recurring intestinal pain and diarrhea. Checking her history, the doctor determined that similar complaints had been recorded and treated during the previous two years. After an examination, she made a tentative diagnosis of an irritable bowel. She prescribed muscle relaxants and told Marilyn to schedule a barium enema. If the symptoms responded to the medication, she could cancel the enema, but if they persisted, she wanted to proceed with the test to rule out other, more serious causes of the problem. Dr. Simon did not elaborate to Marilyn on what those other causes might be.

Taking the advice of a friend, who stressed how unpleasant and inconvenient the procedure was, Marilyn decided not to schedule it but instead to see how the symptoms responded to the medication. Besides, each of the previous incidents had cleared up.

Marilyn, an active athlete, took the muscle relaxants for several days, but she found they made her slightly dizzy and disoriented. She worried about the effect that taking the medication would have on hard exercise. After almost a week, during which the symptoms did not abate, she called the HMO again and spoke to the nurse practitioner in Dr. Simon's office, expressing two concerns: she asked about the side effects of the muscle relaxants and whether competitive athletics were dangerous for her. She also asked for more information about the barium enema, realizing she did not want to undergo an unpleasant procedure without knowing more about what it was supposed to accomplish. She was told that the doctor would call her to answer her questions.

Several days passed without a call from Dr. Simon. Angry by now, Marilyn stopped taking the medication, which continued to bother her, and tried a new over-the-counter antacid. Her symptoms suddenly started to improve, and she did not bother to place a second call to Dr. Simon's office.

A week later, Marilyn realized she had never received a return phone call from Dr. Simon. She reflected angrily on having to take her care into her own hands, but she also realized that had she not done so, she might still be taking a medication that was unpleasant and apparently ineffective. Further, she realized that she could have experienced the discomfort of a procedure that turned out to be unnecessary. Meanwhile, neither her physician nor the nurse practitioner in the practice learned that her symptoms had cleared up.

◆　◆　◆　◆　◆　◆　◆

In all three of these clinical examples, care was suboptimal. Patients in obvious need were ignored, even though in two cases the patients were present in the physician's office and their distress was visible to clinical staff. In one case, the patient's regular physician apparently thought her relationship with her patient was not worth the extra time it would have taken to express her concern, reassure her young patient that a colleague on call that evening would take good care of her, and invite her to call with questions or if any problems developed.

In our view, all three examples represent the failure of individual clinical staff to respond appropriately to patients. More important, however, is the failure of managers—in concert with each plan's doctors—to establish policies and standard practices to ensure that patients are treated not just as a set of presenting symptoms, but as individuals. It appears that the only real harm in these instances was the undermining of patients' confidence in their physicians and in the organizations responsible for their clinical care (in the case of the young softball player, the incident also led to the family's leaving the HMO). Conversely, if such situations are repeated, it is only a matter of time before a patient does suffer avoidable harm.

In the next story, the patient was pleased with the medical care she received but very unhappy with her treatment by clerks over the issue of an erroneous bill.

◆  ◆  ◆  ◆  ◆  ◆  ◆

## Paying the Bill

A young professional woman, Joan West, was cooking alone in her suburban New England home one summer evening. Heating some oil on the stove, her attention was diverted for a moment and the oil burst into flames. She turned off the stove, but as she grabbed for the pot flames shot up her arm, causing her to drop the pot on the floor. Although the fire dissipated quickly, she had painful second-degree burns on her hand and arm and third-degree burns on her leg where the oil had splattered on its way to the floor.

Unable to drive, Joan had the presence of mind to call 911. A few minutes later, an ambulance arrived and drove her the two miles to the closest emergency room, where she was taken into an examining room immediately. There, her hand, arm, and leg were wrapped in large dressings. She was given instructions about how to care for herself for the next several days, during which time she was expected to stay relatively immobile. She was also told that the wounds would need to be checked and the dressings changed daily as the healing process began.

Since Joan and her husband were covered by a network-model HMO, the next morning she called her primary care physician. She explained the situation, asked the doctor to authorize the services she had already used, and tried to make an appointment to have the dressings changed. The primary care physician did authorize the prior services and provided the names of several surgeons affiliated with the same HMO network to change the dressings and provide ongoing treatment of the wounds.

Over the next several weeks, the surgeon saw Joan a number of times, at first daily, then less often as the blisters on her arm were lanced, cleaned, dressed, and began to heal. In due course, she returned to her normal activities with a minimum of scarring, owing to the good and timely treatment she received.

Eventually bills arrived from the hospital indicating that the emergency-room charges had been paid by the HMO minus only the $25 deductible. Joan and her husband were thinking that this new HMO, which they had joined with some trepidation, had turned out to be pretty good. It had taken care of what was obviously justified out-of-plan use with a minimum of hassle and had even responded appropriately, they thought, when another ER visit was needed because none of the surgeons in the network was available on short notice to change the dressing on the first day after the accident.

Then a bill came from the ambulance service for the full amount of the two-mile trip to the hospital ER. Assuming that this was just a minor glitch in the system, Joan called and explained to the clerk at the ambulance service that the ambulance ride should be a covered service authorized by the primary care physician. With that knowledge, the clerk appeared satisfied, saying he would resubmit the bill to the HMO. Joan heard no more about it until—more than a year later—she began to get calls from a billing service in Dallas, which the ambulance company had retained to "straighten out its accounts receivable." She was told there was no record to indicate that the primary care physician had authorized the use of the ambulance, and the HMO refused to pay the bill.

More than a year after sustaining serious burns, Joan was being dunned by the ambulance service even though the HMO had already paid for two emergency-room visits, which had been authorized by the same physician who would have needed to approve the ambulance use. Even though the HMO acknowledged that the incident had justified the (much higher) charges of the ER, it refused to pay the claim for the ambulance that took her there. No one argued that the service was unnecessary or inappropriate or that the patient had had an alternative, only that the ambulance authorization was not in the record. The payment was being denied solely because authorization had not been received within the required forty-eight-hour period.

Eventually, the plan did pay, but only after the benefits manager at the large company the patient worked for—an important customer—intervened. Thus, it was only in response to the benefits manager's "clout" that the HMO finally paid the bill.

◆　◆　◆　◆　◆　◆　◆

The point of this story is that a health care organization's service extends beyond the clinical episode itself; patients can become very dissatisfied even when the clinical service is more than adequate. In this case, the issue for the HMO's clerk on the other end of the phone was not whether the patient's condition required an ambulance or, more generally, how to make a customer feel good about her choice of insurance company in a fiercely competitive market; what mattered to the clerk was whether the proper forms had been filled out in the allotted time. Managers should have had policies in place to prevent an incident like this from ever getting to the point that the customer needed to call her company's benefits manager to resolve it.

## Evidence of Problems: The Physician's Role

The behavior of individuals working for large organizations like the ones in these vignettes is a by-product of the growing "corporatization of health care" (Eckholm, 1994, p. 34). Against such a backdrop, those who rely on organizations for their care—whether it is a managed care company or a walk-in clinic—need more than ever to be able to depend on their professional physician, who they hope is still guided primarily by a professional code of ethics instead of the economic power of his or her employer. Some commentators have expressed concern that the physician's commitment to his or her patients is compromised by the financial arrangements with the organization (Gray, 1991; Rodwin, 1993). They wonder about a physician's ability to be the patient's advocate when the employing or contracting organization is owned by investors seeking a profit, or when regardless of the organization's ownership the physician's compensation increases because he or she sees more patients (is more "productive") and provides fewer services (is more "efficient"). This concern persists, even though some studies show that while they think they are working harder (and may, in fact, be putting in longer hours), physicians in staff-model HMOs actually see fewer patients than their colleagues in fee-for-service practice (Willke & Cotter, 1989). As these concerns suggest, financial incentives create conflicts of interest for physicians in both fee-for-service and other compensation arrangements and in both investor-owned and not-for-profit organizations.

Randall Bock wrote that the management of the franchised, fee-for-service walk-in clinic in which he practiced "tried to keep the charges to patients higher than necessary, and . . . I was finally dismissed for not generating enough charges per patient" (Bock, 1988, p. 785). Patients enjoy the accessibility of clinics in which waiting times are generally short and in which acute but relatively minor illnesses are accommodated well. Doctors also like the clinics, for their simplicity and the reduced intrusion of the business aspects of medicine. But there is a downside, which the following excerpt from Bock's *New England Journal of Medicine* article discusses.

◆ ◆ ◆ ◆ ◆ ◆ ◆

## How Much Is Enough?

"Total revenue is of course the product of the number of patients and the average charge per patient. The number of patients is the less controllable variable. . . . Therefore, many of the staff's—and corporation's—hopes for 'better numbers' rely on increasing the charges per patient, something that, short of increasing prices, can only be achieved by performing more tests or upgrading the charge for office visits. With staff bonuses and morale hanging in the balance, some doctors feel pressured to keep charges up. . . .

"The corporate predilection for testing was expressed in the idea that routine diagnoses should be accompanied by routine tests (and x-ray examinations). These tests, once defined from above as routine, could then be ordered by the nursing staff before the doctor saw the patient. . . . Doctors reluctant to allow nurses this privilege were to be reported to the regional medical director, according to a corporate memo circulated to nurses. . . .

"I am neither absolutist nor doctrinaire in avoiding laboratory tests. Like all clinicians, I order my share of X-ray films that I know will be negative, of cultures whose outcome will not necessarily change my treatment, and so forth. A test can be reassuring in its negativity and can reinforce the need for compliance when it is positive. By a standard of absolute necessity, I order too much. By the corporation's financial formulas, of course, I did not order enough.

"There was neither implicit nor explicit criticism of the quality of my professional care, as it was explained to me. A 'bottom-line' financial assessment had merely been made. Another, more satisfactory doctor in my place would have had a lower threshold for testing and would have generated more money for the corporation. . . .

"The ethos of medicine and the nature of its primary concern—human health and emotions—make medicine a commodity less amenable to harsh business realities than other economic goods such as automobiles, hair spray, or lumber. The question therefore arises, not whether a corporation is doing good business, but whether it is giving medicine and physicians proper respect when it considers a doctor's pricing profile in its decisions on hiring and continued employment" (Bock, 1988, pp. 785–787).

◆  ◆  ◆  ◆  ◆  ◆  ◆

The following vignette presents an excerpt from a recent article by another primary care physician in which he discussed the additional tasks required of primary care physicians in MCOs, as well as the conditions imposed by those organizations on the physicians.

◆ ◆ ◆ ◆ ◆ ◆ ◆

## The Power of the Organization

"[The growth of managed care] contracting has put pressure on primary care physicians to practice as gatekeepers and to participate in various schemes of capitation in which they are put at financial risk. Gatekeeping is not expected from any other physician group, and capitation with risk assumption infrequently involves other specialties.

"Gatekeeping and capitation make expenditures more predictable and profits more certain for insurers. . . . The gatekeeping physician replaces much of the carrier's review function. . . . While enhancing the financial well-being of the carrier, the nonsalaried primary care physician frequently faces relatively low income at the outset and substantial obstacles to fee increases, even when necessary to simply cover increased office expenses. . . .

"In addition, when carriers control the choice of physician for large numbers of patients, they are able to impose nonnegotiable and sometimes onerous contractual terms. Financial and clinical independence for primary care physicians have concurrently eroded" (Alper, 1994, pp. 1523–1524).

◆ ◆ ◆ ◆ ◆ ◆ ◆

Regardless of the financial arrangements, a physician needs a certain amount of time to discover enough about the patient's condition and relevant circumstances to be an effective advocate, not to mention to provide adequate medical care. Yet, as the following commentary makes clear, the trend is toward shorter visits.

◆ ◆ ◆ ◆ ◆ ◆ ◆

## The Doctor's Time with Patients

In a letter to *The New York Times,* a midwestern physician lamented the focus on costs and complained that little attention is paid to the doctor-patient relationship even though it is "the hallmark of high-quality American medicine." He argued that it must be preserved.

"In a single brief encounter with a physician, a patient is given a diagnosis—usually the comforting news that nothing is seriously wrong. Concerns about the origin of symptoms, the natural history of the illness, and implications for family members are addressed. Guilt and worry are alleviated. All of this is efficiently done in 15 minutes in the United States in most primary care settings.

"All national surveys suggest that people in the United States want more, not less, time with their physicians. But if economics alone drives new managed care plans, administrators will press for the least number of physicians per 1,000 enrolled patients. There will be pressure to see more patients in less time. . . .

"In the context of the physician-patient relationship, face to face time with a physician is both access and quality. If it is reduced, both access and quality are reduced, and the possibility exists that overall cost will increase as unattended illnesses become more severe and expensive to treat.

"It seems to me we should measure and publish average direct, patient-physician times for all approved health care plans. Such times with patients should be rewarded financially and be promoted as a criterion for quality health care" (Wenzel, 1994, p. 16).

◆ ◆ ◆ ◆ ◆ ◆ ◆

Moreover, physicians are concerned with more than just policies limiting the amount of time they can spend with patients, as the next two examples illustrate.

◆ ◆ ◆ ◆ ◆ ◆ ◆

## The Rigidity of Company Policies

A managed care plan has a policy that implanting new shunts in patients' arms for dialysis must be done on an outpatient basis; the policy refuses to pay for overnight stays. When physicians call the managed care company asking for permission to keep a patient in the hospital overnight, the clerk on the other end of the line (who may or may not have clinical training or experience) routinely denies the request because of the company's policy.

While that policy may be appropriate for many patients, some—and not only those who are elderly—do not heal well and are at risk for bleeding and infection. Their special characteristics make the general policy inappropriate for them; as a result, they should be kept in the hospital for a night and sometimes longer. The doctor faces several choices, none of them good: send the patient home, knowing the risk, and hope for the best; appeal the clerk's ruling, which is time-consuming and is not resolved until well after the overnight stay; or keep the patient in the hospital because it is indicated medically, knowing that the hospital stay will not be covered by the plan.

♦  ♦  ♦  ♦  ♦  ♦  ♦

One consideration in decision making, as illustrated in the following excerpt from a letter to *The New York Times*, is the risk that the patient will develop complications after having been discharged from care because of an MCO's policies and will sue the physician for malpractice.

♦  ♦  ♦  ♦  ♦  ♦  ♦

### Prior Authorization

"The law holds the physician responsible for decisions made by the managed care company. My greatest fear as a psychiatrist is that a suicidal patient will come to my office and need more visits than the managed care company allows. I can petition the decision, but the company may not allow me to see the patient more frequently.

"If patients should then harm themselves or anyone else, I am the one sued, not the managed care company. Contracts between managed care companies and physicians not only absolve the companies of clinical responsibility but also allow them to dismiss from their list of providers doctors who get sued" (Becker, 1994, p. 8).

◆  ◆  ◆  ◆  ◆  ◆  ◆

The increasing tendency of MCOs to install prior-authorization requirements to govern decisions about care means that the treatment may be determined not by the physician in the examining room with the patient but by a clerk on the other end of a telephone line. In that case, the role of the doctor is to recommend and request authorization for the treatment, while the clerk, usually relying on a set of written protocols, either grants or denies the request. Besides their complaints about who is in the best position to know what the patient needs, physicians are also concerned about their liability, even when their recommendation is rejected by the organization's representative.

Although we did not confirm the validity of all of the specific claims made in the stories in this chapter, it appears reasonable to us to conclude that even many clinicians who concede the need to be efficient and to contain spending are concerned that some of the cuts being made are affecting the adequacy of the care being provided in a variety of institutions throughout the country. The fundamental business of these organizations is to deliver health care services to people who need them. Since they operate under onerous constraints, especially in very competitive markets, the doctors who deliver those services will need to make different clinical decisions than they would if money were no object. The issue illustrated in these examples is that managers who impose rigid rules on physicians (for example, protocols that deny the physician the ability to decide that a particular patient needs to stay overnight) in order to accomplish the purpose of delivering good care efficiently risk the resistance and hostility of physicians, the dissatisfaction of patients, and, in some instances, avoidable medical accidents or injuries. The better alternative, which we elaborate later in the book, is for managers to engage physicians both to develop policies and procedures that enable them to deliver good care without wasting resources and to create an organizational culture that values both quality and efficiency.

The contemporary medical care arena in the United States has elevated the importance of health care organizations not only because of potential efficiencies. Organizations also have the capacity to manage the *processes* of care better than individual clinicians practicing in the fragmented, decentralized medical care system many of us grew up with. But physicians—and managers—often do not understand either the potential for better management of medical services or how to maximize it.

◆ ◆ ◆ ◆ ◆ ◆ ◆

## Failing to Take Advantage of the Organization's Resources

The obstetric department in a staff-model HMO had been feeling the pressures of increased patient care demands and tighter resources. One physician had recently resigned and although hiring was a high priority, no replacements were in sight.

One of the obstetricians, Dr. Williams, had been looking forward to her vacation for months. To prepare, she arranged coverage for her office practice, and the HMO arranged coverage for her labor and delivery duty. The day before her departure, she examined a woman who was in her ninth week of pregnancy but who had been spotting. Tests confirmed that the pregnancy was no longer viable, and Dr. Williams attempted to schedule the woman that afternoon for a D&C. When she found that the OR was booked, she informed the patient that her procedure would be scheduled for the first day after her vacation.

The next evening, the patient began to bleed heavily and to experience severe pain. She went to the emergency room, where the ER physicians were shocked to hear that her D&C had been put off for a week. They performed the procedure, but they also called Jane Henning, the administrator of the ob/gyn department, who was equally concerned when she heard the story. Jane was upset that the patient's physician had not asked her to try to get the procedure scheduled more appropriately and she was sure that if she herself had been involved, it could have been arranged.

When Dr. Williams returned from her vacation, she explained to Jane that all the other physicians in the practice were already feeling overworked and she did not see a way for the procedure to be scheduled sooner. She explained that she had joined an HMO to avoid that kind of conflict and the need "to hassle with" the arrangements to solve it. She did not seem to understand the inconsistency in her behavior: the HMO could not solve the problem for her if she did not at least take the time to bring it to the attention of appropriate staff.

❖ ❖ ❖ ❖ ❖ ❖ ❖ ❖

The increasingly competitive medical care environment brings new obligations for physicians to be cost conscious, but practicing in organizations also introduces increased *opportunities* for them to provide good service. Perhaps these opportunities are not maximized for the benefit of patients because doctors do not always recognize them, or perhaps doctors do not understand the full extent of their professional obligations in the new health care world.

The previous example tells a story in which the quality of the patient's care was compromised by a physician who not only did not advocate for her patient but also did not attempt to mobilize the added resources available in a staff-model HMO that might not be present in office-based private practice. The manager was ready—and probably able—to support the physician's clinical judgment, but the physician did not recognize that being in a staff-model HMO can have advantages and that she need not shoulder the entire burden of arranging care for her patient.

Another example involving the ob/gyn department of a staff-model HMO, one with a national reputation for its innovations in data collection and management, shows that managers and doctors alike have not learned what is optimal behavior in a complex medical care organization.

◆  ◆  ◆  ◆  ◆  ◆  ◆

## Duplicate Records

The obstetrician/gynecologists learned from experience not to rely on the data system for reports about abnormal Pap smears. Multiple reports were often received, and sometimes none came. Virtually all of the department's physicians compensated for this uncertainty by maintaining in their own offices parallel manual files with Pap smear results. Keeping the files up to date and organizing them so they would know when to schedule the next test took a significant amount of physician time, but the physicians told themselves it was necessary to do so in order to be confident that they knew the condition of their patients. Of course, the time the physicians spent on these records came from somewhere—either from uncompensated personal time, which tended to increase their frustration, anger, and distance from an organization they felt failed to support them adequately; or from compensated work time, which reduced the time they had available for their patients.

◆  ◆  ◆  ◆  ◆  ◆  ◆

In this instance, physicians did not feel that managers supported them appropriately by creating and operating a clinical data base that could serve physicians and patients. As a result, the HMO was not realizing the benefits of automation in the daunting effort to organize and thereby gain a measure of control over the complexity of modern medical care. At the same time, instead of bringing the problem to the managers so it could be solved to everyone's benefit, the physicians crafted a solution that failed to recognize the heavy resource costs in time spent maintaining a dual file, a cost they bore on their own shoulders. The physicians' "solution" added to the HMO's costs because physician time had to be allotted to manage the lab results. Experiences such as this may go a long way toward explaining why managers believe doctors do not work hard enough if they do not see "enough" patients, while at the same time doctors believe they are working harder than ever and enjoying it less.

The stakes and the professional responsibilities are high, and part of the challenge for physicians is to learn how to be effective members of an organization. If physicians who attempt to goad the organization into functioning better find that the managers they are dealing with do not respond appropriately to requests for better information, then they must demand satisfaction from more-senior managers, who may have a better appreciation of the high stakes involved. In any event, the physician's ultimate responsibility is to provide good care for the patient. The organization's failure to support the physician in the effort to do so may mean not only that the physician is compromised vis-à-vis the patient, but also that the strain of continually "fighting the system" will take a toll on both the physician, who may disengage psychologically or leave altogether, and the organization, which will be less efficient, less effective, and less satisfying to subscribers.

A final story raises the issue of defining the boundaries of the clinician role in an organizational context.

◆  ◆  ◆  ◆  ◆  ◆  ◆

## Whose Responsibility Is It?

An elderly widow, who was independent and proud of being able to take care of herself, was discharged to her home after a hospital stay, still weak and somewhat disoriented. Her granddaughter picked her up from the hospital and took her to the apartment she lived in alone. Her son, who was self-employed with a flexible schedule, dropped by in the afternoon to visit and was concerned that his mother would have difficulty caring for herself, for a few days at least and perhaps longer. He arranged for an aide from a home health agency to bathe her, help her to the bathroom, and prepare some of her meals. The family did the grocery shopping, and either her son or one of her college-age grandchildren visited at least once each day and were in touch by phone. No one at the hospital, a major teaching institution in a large city, even asked questions about how she would manage while she regained her strength at home.

◆　◆　◆　◆　◆　◆

The last three vignettes are examples of what may be a growing tendency: some health care professionals who work in organizations appear to regard themselves as employees governed more by the policies and interests of the distant organization than by the service-oriented standards of their professions. One implication is that they shift some of the physician's obligation to care for the patient to the organization; the result may be that patients receive suboptimal care because of the organization's inadequacies even though the individual clinicians have done the best they can. It's the organization's fault!

In the story "Failing to Take Advantage of the Organization's Resources," a doctor tried to cope with what she thought were organization-inspired limitations by postponing a patient's treatment in spite of the risk to the patient's health. She did not put her duty to her patient above other concerns. In "Duplicate Records," instead of insisting that the organization perform better, the obstetricians bore the cost (which they probably did not recognize as a cost, but certainly resented) of creating a parallel manual information system for Pap smear results. The individual clinical staff in "Whose Responsibility Is It?" acted as if their obligation began when the patient entered the examining room and ended when she left the hospital. No one involved in the patient's hospital care thought about how she would cope once she left the hospital. And the managers responsible for the organization either had not created a process for developing policies that would support a broader definition of their obligation to patients or were not ensuring the quality of the services provided by hospital personnel.

Undoubtedly, these tendencies are reinforced by financial considerations dictated by insurance policies that exclude most non-hospital, nonmedical services in an increasingly money-conscious, competitive marketplace. They occur even though patients who fail to get the supportive services they need following an illness are at greater risk of relapse and rehospitalization, which requires additional expenditures on the part of the insurer. But that is only part of a syndrome that is creating a cohort of demoralized physicians and a deprofessionalized workplace that encourages a "time clock" mentality instead of celebrating the physicians'—and now the health care organization's—ethical commitments to their patients. As we have tried to make clear, the stakes are high and the challenge to both professions—medicine and management—is great.

## Facing the Situation

We do not on the one hand mean to suggest with these true stories that all of today's health care organizations are uniformly uncaring bureaucracies with no commitment to patient service, or that today's health care professionals are no longer guided by the principles of medical ethics. On the other hand, it would be naïve of us to ignore the powerful force that financial incentives exert on provider behavior and on the professionals' attachment, whether through contract or employment, to large, growing health care organizations that may understand their power better than their responsibilities.

Nonetheless, the corporatization of health care is a fact of life and its continuing growth, which may be inevitable, has its champions. Kenneth Abramowitz, a market analyst in New York, is quoted by *The New York Times* as saying, "And what's wrong with that? Corporations produce hotel rooms and toothpaste and automobiles, and the country does fine. You still have to produce a service and monitor and improve it, for a finite price" (Eckholm, 1994, p. 34). As these vignettes demonstrate, many health care organizations may not yet be oriented primarily to producing quality service or to monitoring and improving it. Yet unless they learn to do better, everyone will suffer. Those who champion market forces as the ultimate arbiter expect competition to drive out the bad companies and assure the success of the good ones. Companies that do not satisfy will fail because customers will desert them and flock to those offering better services at more reasonable prices, and the public will be the ultimate beneficiary. This logic assumes that in each market some companies indeed do a terrific job, while others are driven by their determination not just to emulate those exemplars but to surpass them (or at least to avoid failure). But what if none of the companies—or only a few—really "has it right"? Even though some dedicated individuals provide technically excellent, caring service to patients, they may do so not because the organizations have created conditions that facilitate and reward such behavior but because they are driven by other standards, perhaps the ethics of their professions. Their colleagues down the hall may be more ordinary. The problem is that *to succeed, an organization must be better than its competitors—even if only a little better.* If the organizations, as organizations, do not know how to produce good quality care reliably, and if they as well as the caregivers who work under their auspices have other motivations besides providing good service, then we should all be concerned. Indeed, some of those who are poorly served by the organization may be harmed. Health care is not toothpaste! The stakes in the health care market can be life itself.

Health care organizations and the financial constraints under which they operate are here to stay. Even if we wanted to, we could not defeat them. Therefore, they must be improved. In our view, a prime reason for the failure of health care organizations to reach a uniformly high standard of service is that managers have not learned how to engage physicians and other health care professionals as partners in that quest. Many, if not most, do not even recognize that as their role or task. And physicians have not learned to ask for—or, if necessary, to demand—the administrative support they and their patients need. Yet, we also believe (although it is harder to demonstrate) that the care provided in or through organizations can be technically better than and at least equally caring as the best care provided in the days when medicine was a cottage industry. Neither managers nor physicians appear to recognize that organizations have advantages for patients and for delivering good quality care, much less know how to maximize them.

With this book we hope to make a contribution to changing that reality. Our focus is on what happens *after* the managed care contract has been signed. How is care delivered? How are patients served? How can the advantages of organizations be brought to bear on the challenges facing modern medicine? If nothing else, we hope to persuade health care managers and physicians that the best hope for the future depends on mutual partnership in pursuit of effective care efficiently delivered.

# 2

## Our Growing Dependence on Organizations

### HMOs, PPOs, and Everything in Between

The health care system is changing in ways that have important implications for the future, and health care organizations are at the center of this turbulence. In earlier times, the image of health care in the minds of most Americans was that of a longtime community resident visiting the family doctor at his small office for services provided by the physician himself and perhaps his nurse. Indeed, sometimes the kindly physician visited his bedridden patient at home.

By contrast, today growing numbers of Americans in a much more mobile society are turning to organizations for their care, which has become technically more complex and often involves many different people with a variety of capabilities. Moreover, growing numbers and proportions of clinicians are working in or under the aegis of organizations.

Public debates about the health care system tend to concentrate on the insurance dimension, obscuring this more critical phenomenon: that organizations have become so prominent in the delivery of health care services that they are now the mainstream of American medicine. This state has emerged only gradually as the result of an accumulation of decisions by individuals and organizations in response to the changing pressures they faced. The result is that we are only now able to acknowledge the magnitude of this new dependence, to try to understand its implications, and to master the challenges and opportunities that it presents to us.

In Chapters Two through Four, we lay the groundwork for our later argument about the physician-manager partnership by demonstrating (1) the magnitude of the organizational dimension of the U.S. health care system and (2) the need to understand better the complex relations between managers and physicians. Here, in Chapter Two, we define the organizational component in the health services sector and provide measures of both its size and its astonishing growth. The two chapters that follow discuss the relationships among four important participant groups in the health care sector: citizens and employers, on the purchasing side of the equation (Chapter Three); and physicians and managers, on the delivery end (Chapter Four).

## Dimensions of the Organizational Component in the Health Care Sector

We believe that the extent to which the health care system succeeds in meeting the challenge of providing effective care efficiently to all Americans will *depend* on the nature of the influence that managers of health care organizations (hospitals, HMOs, PPOs, and PHOs, among others) exert on physicians and other clinicians. The reason is simple: more and more Americans rely on organizations for their care, and more and more physicians practice their profession under the banner of organizations. In this chapter, we demonstrate the astounding prominence in the United States of several of the most important types of health care organizations.

The presence of organizations in health care is not new. But until recently, almost all were either hospitals, which provided certain services to patients who remained overnight in a hospital bed, or insurance companies, which paid bills for certain (usually the expensive) services. Neither type of organization was much concerned about the cost of services a patient received because, first, the hospital as well as the patient's doctors earned their income by collecting payments for each service provided; and second, the insurers paid whatever bills were submitted to them, usually raising the following year's premium in order to maintain the desired level of profit or surplus.

Now, however, by *organization* we mean not only hospitals and insurers but also HMOs, PPOs, other managed care arrangements, PHOs, integrated service networks (ISNs), storefront clinics, multispecialty group practices, nursing homes, and others. Yet our dependence on organizations does not mean that people necessarily go to receive or provide care in a large building housing many clinicians. In fact, today's organization can include the same private doctors practicing in the same small offices with the same patients that they have been seeing for years. The difference is that now the organization—whether simply a payer of services or, like an HMO or hospital, a provider—operates under a set of *financial constraints*, which give it a much stronger stake than previously in the care delivered by its clinicians, including physicians who practice off-site in their own offices.

Ultimately, what is at stake for the organization is its very survival. In a competitive environment, the organization must be concerned that unless its actions satisfy the "customers"—both patients and the clinicians who provide care—it will lose them to competitors. For that reason, managers, who are the organization's custodians, must assure themselves *both* that clinicians are responsive to patients' felt needs for services, and that in meeting those needs the clinicians not only provide effective care but also pay attention to the cost of the services they provide or order. Failure to do so can mean, in the first case, that dissatisfied patients will seek others to provide their care, and in the second, that financially conscious subscribers will shop for a lower-cost alternative. Managers must also satisfy the organization's physicians because otherwise they may leave, perhaps taking patients with them. The physicians may undermine the organization's goals through their control of the clinical function, or they may organize as adversaries of management in order to gain concessions on issues that are important to them. These observations hold equally for all health care organizations, although the particular manifestations vary by type of organization. Most of the rest of this book concerns the relationships between managers, who have responsibility for their organizations' survival, and physicians, who have responsibility for their patients' care. Our goals are to understand, first, the institutional contexts in which managers and physicians operate, including evidence that neither they nor their health care organizations are performing optimally; and second, the tasks they perform, the factors that motivate them, and the opportunities for improving their performance (and that of their organizations). An additional objective is to provide guidance to both managers and doctors on how to achieve the partnership we believe is necessary in the modern health care environment.

Before getting to those issues, in the rest of this chapter we sketch the dimensions of the organizational component of the health care system, primarily by discussing three of the most important types of organizations on the contemporary scene: hospitals, HMOs, and PPOs.

## Hospitals

For most of the past hundred years or more, the hospital has been the primary health care organization in the United States. Hospitals began as facilities for the sick poor who had no families to care for them. In an era in which medicine had limited powers to cure illness, most very sick people stayed at home and received care from family and occasionally from doctors who visited them there. The distinctive role of the modern hospital, in contrast, has been to provide inpatient care for very sick people who need either surgery or other services that cannot be provided elsewhere (for example, isolation because patients are susceptible to infections, or close monitoring because they have high fevers and are in debilitated states).

Although it remains a large and important part of the health care system, in recent years, the character and role of the hospital sector have changed dramatically. Some of this change is reflected in the statistics in Table 2.1.

Between 1972 and 1992, the number of hospitals, number of hospital beds, and occupancy rates all declined. In 1992, there were 530 fewer hospitals than in 1972, a drop of 8.6 percent, although the number increased in the early part of the period before beginning a steady decline.[1] The number of hospital beds declined by only 1.1 percent; but again because of an increase during the first part of the period, that figure masks much more dramatic recent reductions. In seven short years at the end of that period, from the peak in 1985 to 1992, more than 100,000 hospital beds were taken out of service, heralding the reversal of a long-standing trend. Most importantly for the future, occupancy rates declined from 76.1 percent in 1972 to 66.6 percent in 1992, even though the number of beds declined and the bed-to-population ratio also declined.[2]

Far from meaning that the hospital has lost its importance, however, these trends signify that its role in the medical care system has been changing. Patients admitted to hospital beds today tend to be sicker on average than previously. Perhaps even more significant, hospitals have become much more important as providers of outpatient services. The latter point can be seen from the figures in Table 2.1, which show that in the same twenty-year period during which inpatient capacity and services were declining so dramatically, outpatient visits almost doubled and emergency-department visits increased by 59 percent. Finally, reflecting both the changes in role and the growth in certain administrative functions, the number of hospital employees (that is, full-time equivalents, or FTEs) *grew* by 72 percent. That increase and the more-than-doubling of FTEs per 100 patients are indicators that the work of hospitals in 1992 was very different from the work of their 1972 counterparts.

These changes have two principal causes. First, advances in medical science—powerful new drugs and laser and laparoscopic

Table 2.1. Short-Stay Hospitals, Selected Statistics, 1972–1992.

| Ownership | 1972 | 1992 | Percent Change 1972–1992 |
|---|---|---|---|
| Number of Hospitals | | | |
| Federal | 401 | 325 | −19.0 |
| Nonprofit | 3,301 | 3,173 | −3.9 |
| Proprietary | 738 | 723 | −20.0 |
| State/local | 1,707 | 1,396 | −18.2 |
| Total | 6,147 | 5,617 | −8.6 |
| Number of Beds (000s) | | | |
| Federal | 143 | 89 | −37.8 |
| Nonprofit | 617 | 656 | + 6.3 |
| Proprietary | 57 | 99 | +73.7 |
| State/local | 205 | 167 | −18.5 |
| Total | 1,022 | 1,011 | − 1.1 |
| Occupancy Rate (Percent) | | | |
| Federal | 80.0 | 77.3 | −2.7 |
| Nonprofit | 77.5 | 67.9 | −9.6 |
| Proprietary | 68.7 | 52.0 | −16.7 |
| State/local | 71.0 | 64.7 | − 6.3 |
| Total | 76.1 | 66.6 | −9.5 |
| Visits to All Hospitals (Millions) | | | |
| Outpatient Visits | 219.2 | 417.9 | +90.6 |
| ER Visits | 60.1 | 95.8 | +59.4 |
| Personnel (000s) | | | |
| Federal | 232 | 306 | +31.9 |
| Nonprofit | 1,473 | 2,692 | +82.8 |
| Proprietary | 105 | 285 | +171.4 |
| State/local | 473 | 643 | +35.9 |
| Total | 2,283 | 3,926 | +72.0 |
| FTE/100 patients | 221 | 525 | +137.6 |

Source: Adapted from Statistical Abstract of the U.S., 1994, Table 179, p. 125.

surgery, for example—have made it possible for patients to recover more quickly than previously and in some cases to avoid hospitalization altogether. Similarly, new surgical techniques and local anesthetics have made it possible to perform many procedures on outpatients, who might arrive at a hospital in the early morning for a procedure that takes perhaps two hours, spend most of the day in a recovery room, and return home before the end of the day, thus avoiding an overnight hospital stay. In some cases, these procedures are done in surgical centers that are not connected with hospitals, but many are done in new outpatient surgery facilities located in the hospital building.

Second, changes in the financing of medical care have given hospitals a powerful reason to introduce new drugs, surgical techniques, and other technical advances that have made it possible to avoid hospitalization in many cases and to shorten stays in others. Beginning in the late 1960s and early 1970s, the health care system as a whole, and hospitals in particular, have been preoccupied with health care expenditures.

For good reason. From 1970 through 1992, personal health care expenditures grew from $64.8 billion to $782.5 billion, an increase of more than 1,100 percent (Levit et al., 1994). This growth coincided with the expansion of third-party payment, which made it possible for most Americans to avail themselves of the benefits of modern medicine during a period that saw both unprecedented innovation and dramatic increases in the probability of benefiting from medical care.

The prodigious growth in spending created a mounting burden for payers (especially employers and the federal government), which pressured providers, including hospitals, to cut their costs and charges. So, while hospitals remained an important organizational form in the health care system, they adapted to increased pressures in the health care environment by changing their role. Concurrently, in response to some of the same pressures, other organizational forms expanded and became even more prominent in the health care system; in addition, wholly new organizational types were created. Chief among the former is the expanding variety of HMOs; the latter include other types of MCOs, such as PPOs.

We turn now to brief discussions of each.

## Health Maintenance Organizations

In 1973, not long after the term "health maintenance organization" was coined, Roemer and Shonick described the HMO concept as requiring "the assumption of responsibility for the health of a population by an organized entity, in consideration of a fixed, prepaid amount of money" (Roemer & Shonick, 1973, p. 271). They went on to define an HMO as an organization that:

(a) makes a contract with consumers (or employers on their behalf) to assure the delivery of stated health services of measurable quality;

(b) has an enrolled population;

(c) offers a stated broad range of personal health service benefits, including at least physician services and hospital care;

(d) is paid on an advance capitation basis [Roemer & Shonick, 1973, p. 272].

In the intervening years, as HMOs have grown in numbers, they have also come to encompass several varieties, usually referred to as the following four "models":

1. Staff: "an organization that employs and controls physicians directly and pays them salary" (Welch, Hillman, & Pauly, 1990, p. 221)

2. Group: an organization that contracts with a single physician group practice

3. Network: an organization that contracts with multiple physician groups, often connected with one another through their association with a common hospital

4. Independent practice association (IPA): an organization that contracts with individual physicians in private practices

Although Welch and his colleagues have pointed out the limitations of this typology and have attempted usefully to identify the underlying dimensions on which the several types differ, for present purposes it will suffice. Later, we identify issues concerning the management challenge and manager-physician relationships that vary with the refinements Welch and colleagues introduced.

The number of HMOs grew rapidly until it peaked at 707 in 1987. Since then, the number has been declining steadily and dramatically, primarily as a result of consolidation (Table 2.2). Although the distribution is not uniform, HMOs are a national phenomenon, found in all regions of the country.

Table 2.2. Health Maintenance Organizations, 1988–1993.

|  | Year | | | | | | Percent Change (1988–1993) |
|---|---|---|---|---|---|---|---|
|  | 1988 | 1989 | 1990 | 1991 | 1992 | 1993 |  |
| No. of Plans |  |  |  |  |  |  |  |
| Staff | 61 | 66 | 64 | 59 | 56 | 53 | −13 |
| Group | 85 | 85 | 77 | 73 | 71 | 68 | −20 |
| Network | 106 | 86 | 98 | 84 | 72 | 68 | −36 |
| IPA | 407 | 386 | 371 | 365 | 363 | 351 | −16 |
| Total | 659 | 623 | 610 | 581 | 562 | 540 | −22 |
| Enrollment |  |  |  |  |  |  |  |
| (in 000s) | 33,715 | 35,031 | 37,538 | 40,388 | 44,373 | 48,978 | +45.3 |

*Source:* Adapted from Marion Merrell Dow, *Managed Care Digest: HMO Edition,* 1993 and 1994 reports, p. 7.

The first thing the table indicates is the dominance of IPAs as a type, accounting for 65 percent of all HMOs in 1993. The other three types shared the balance roughly equally (the highest varied by less than 3 percent from the lowest). Second, the table indicates that all four types declined in numbers, demonstrating that the general trend toward consolidation of HMOs is occurring across the board.

Finally, Table 2.2 shows that while the number of HMOs has been declining, the number and share of the population depending on HMOs for their care have been growing dramatically. From 10.8 million subscribers in 1982 (Cherner, 1993, table 3.1.3), the population of HMO enrollees soared to almost 49 million in 1993. Of particular importance for our interest in management, 40.7 percent of subscribers are in IPAs and another 17.2 percent are in mixed plans, largely a combination of network- and IPA-model plans (Cherner, 1993). While the management challenge is substantial in all HMOs, it is greatest in IPAs and mixed plans because in many urban markets physicians tend to have relationships with more than one plan and to have only a fraction of their patients in each. The resultant combination of divided loyalties, multiple information systems each of which has only limited capabilities, and other factors makes it more difficult for managers in those types of HMOs to influence practice patterns of their physicians than is the case for managers in staff- and group-model plans. It is also important to note that one reason physicians and citizens alike prefer IPAs is that they represent the smallest change from previous arrangements. As cost constraints get tighter, however, IPAs will face the challenges we write about even more urgently than other HMO types, and they will have fewer tools to deal with them. As a consequence, they may be especially vulnerable and therefore prone to attempt draconian initiatives in a frantic effort to survive. Under such conditions, we believe there will be much to be concerned about.

Staff- and group-model plans have organizational and financial advantages over the other types of HMOs; they also have many fewer physicians. With six and eight physicians per thousand enrollees in 1991, staff- and group-model plans had only 16 to 29 percent of the physicians-per-thousand figures the other types of plans had (Cherner, 1993, table 3.5.1). Moreover, in the case of network- and IPA-model plans, these figures represent not FTE physicians but the number of different physicians associated with each plan. When the physician-patient relationship is expressed as the number of patients per primary care physician, we can see clearly that the average physician associated with IPAs and networks has 160 and 178 patients respectively, compared to 810 and 704 respectively for staff- and group-model physicians. Because IPA- and network-model physicians are treating other patients as well, their divided loyalties further dilute managerial influence.

Since an HMO's gross income is predetermined by the premiums and the number of subscribers, one of the manager's concerns is that clinicians conserve the resources used in treating patients, for example as measured by costs per thousand subscribers. That goal is much easier to accomplish if the plan has fewer resources to begin with, because a testing machine or a clinician that is present is much easier to use than one that must be found when the need arises. Under those conditions, the temptation to use an available resource may be great while the barriers to using it are low. Thus, since IPAs and network HMOs tend to offer many physicians to their subscribers, it would not be surprising to find that visit rates per subscriber are higher than in a staff or group model, especially when physicians are paid on a fee-for-service basis and thus earn an additional amount for each visit. By the same token, having fewer available physician-hours with which to serve patients, staff- and group-model HMOs should have lower visit rates. In addition, a manager's attempts to influence large numbers of physicians dispersed in many sites over a wide geographic area will require much more effort and skill than his or her capacity to affect smaller numbers more concentrated in fewer locations or perhaps even at a single site.

## Preferred Provider Organizations

PPOs were invented in the late 1970s and grew to prominence during the 1980s as another response to the increasingly competitive nature of the health care market of that period. The quest was for a new type of plan promising to contain costs on the one hand, while permitting the continuation of fee-for-service medicine and avoiding disruptions of existing patient-physician relationships on the other. The PPO device was an insurance product that called for discounts if patients used physicians, hospitals, and other providers who, because they agreed to accept lower fees, were "preferred" by the insurer. However, patients still had the option of using other providers if they wanted to and were willing to pay a higher price when doing so. Thus when they used providers within the network, as much as 80 percent of the bill might be covered; but if in a particular instance they chose to seek care from another provider, then the insurer would pay perhaps only 60 percent of the bill. The actual payment differentials varied with the plan.

PPOs were popular with physicians because they could continue to receive fees for the services they provided. They were also popular with patients, who retained the comprehensive coverage they had always had and preserved the flexibility to use the system as they chose. Patients were not locked into a set of unfamiliar providers, they had experience with the arrangements for using and paying for services, and the increment in price for leaving the network appeared to be manageable.

Later on, HMOs introduced a variation of this idea: point-of-service (POS) plans. They provided the benefits of HMOs (complete coverage and therefore greater control of service costs by the plan) but avoided the lock-in to particular clinicians by offering subscribers the option of using outside professionals if the subscriber was willing to pay the difference between the HMO's cost for the service and the outside provider's charge.

We include PPOs here for two reasons. First, they have proved to be quite popular. From 1984 through 1992, the number of plans grew from 115 to 1,036 (800 percent), and enrollment from more than 12 million in 1987 to almost 58 million (an increase of 383 percent) only six years later (American Association of Preferred Provider Organizations, personal communication).

Second, because they operate in the same competitive markets as HMOs, PPOs face similar pressures to contain expenditures; therefore, their managers must meet the same challenge to control medical care costs as managers of HMOs do. Although to date the evidence is limited, it appears that these hybrid arrangements have had difficulty controlling expenditures (Miller & Luft, 1993).

## Conclusion

This picture of organizations involved in the delivery of health care services is not complete because it excludes some additional organizational types:

Community health centers

PHOs

ISNs

Long-term care facilities

Hospices

Public health departments

Employee health services available in many large companies

Department of Veterans Affairs' array of health services

CHAMPUS system for military personnel and their families

If we were to present similar data on these organizations and the large number of people who depend on them for either services or their livelihood, we would only strengthen the two primary conclusions of this chapter: (1) the majority of Americans depend on health care organizations for services, and (2) most practitioners provide services under the auspices of one or more health care organizations. Those additional data would reveal a still greater role for organizations in the U.S. health care system.

Nonetheless, extrapolating from the partial picture presented here, we can clearly see the central issue: *given the pervasive influence of organizations in the delivery of care, it is critically important to focus on the efforts of the managers of those institutions to influence the clinicians whose actions determine their viability.* CEOs, medical directors, and others certainly will attempt at the very least to contain the costs associated with delivering services. Good managers will also monitor and attempt to enhance clinician responsiveness to patients and the quality of the services being delivered. But these observations raise other questions, as well:

- To what degree will managers concentrate on cost containment without also attending to access and quality issues?

- What *methods* will they use to attempt to influence clinical decisions?

- Regardless of the explicit focus of their efforts, can the impact on access and quality, as well as on costs, be measured?

- If so, can some organizations be shown to be more effective than others?

- Since each management effort will generate its own costs (which must then be added to the cost of services), can the increments in administrative costs also be measured?

- Assuming these complex activities and outcomes can be measured, will those organizations that invest in improving access, quality, and efficiency be rewarded in the marketplace?

- If not, will they continue to make the investment, or will regulatory methods be needed to focus their efforts on serving subscribers?

- Will the answers to these questions vary by the degree of competitiveness in the local market? By whether the organization operates as a for-profit or not-for-profit entity? By whether it is freestanding or part of a multi-unit chain?

These are some of the questions raised by our growing national dependence on organizations in the delivery of services. While we are not able to answer them in this book, we attempt to put them in clear focus and provide guidance to those who seek empirical answers to them. We believe that these questions are of fundamental importance to the future of the U.S. health care system and that a major investment is needed to find these answers.

In this chapter we have tried to lay important groundwork for what comes next. We have attempted to show that Americans depend on health care organizations to a much larger extent than ever before; that professional caregivers practice as employees of or contractors with organizations much more than previously; and, especially since relevant health system experience is too limited to be much of a guide, that the resulting management challenge confronting these organizations is staggering and varies in important ways with the type of organization being considered.

In the next two chapters, we examine the impact of these changing conditions on four key groups of people: citizens and their employers, who are the primary purchasers of coverage and care; and the providers of the services they purchase: their physicians and the managers of these burgeoning organizations.

3

# The Health Care Customer
## in the New Marketplace

An assessment of any complex social system, especially in a period of great change or when the goal is deliberately to promote change, is aided by a conceptualization of what that system *should* look like if it functioned optimally. With that in mind, we first sketch the relationship between ordinary citizens and their primary care physicians. In doing so, we believe this is what most Americans would like their experience with the health care system to be. Then, we identify some of the factors that make this ideal difficult to achieve in contemporary American society, including the mobility of the population and some of the methods used by employers to try to contain their health care expenditures. The importance of these features of the health care system will be apparent in Chapter Six, where we demonstrate that health care delivered through organizations does not meet either this popular view of what the health care system should be or an ideal to which, in our view, we as a society implicitly aspire.

## Doctor-Patient Relationships

Americans often talk with one another about "their" doctors, using such language as "Who is *your* internist?" "Do your children *have* a pediatrician?" Implicit in these phrases signifying possession of an individual physician is an ongoing relationship between the patient and that physician. The patient has come to know the physician as a result of having consulted him or her over an extended period; similarly, the physician has come to know the patient as an individual who is more than a collection of symptoms presented during an office visit.

The patient and the physician have come to know one another and to respect and trust one another through the shared experience of seeking and providing care. The patient seeks help from the physician when he feels the need, especially when he is ill. In turn, the physician responds promptly with services addressed to the patient's "felt need."

The physician treats the patient appropriately in the course of an illness, and not more aggressively than is warranted to either cure the patient's condition or relieve symptoms. At the same time, he or she recognizes and addresses the patient's anxiety and other feelings about his condition by listening and responding with sensitivity. Over the course of time, as a result of the developing relationship, the patient comes to recognize the limitations of medical care and yet has less anxiety about illness. He does not *demand* treatments he has read about in the popular press or heard about from friends but instead *inquires* about those treatments and accepts the physician's judgment as to their appropriateness.

Finally, the experience out of which this idealized view develops includes the physician's charging relatively modest fees for his services. He does this in part because although practice is his primary means of earning a living, his principal commitment is to *serving* his patients; the service he provides is to a large extent the time he spends listening, giving advice, and prescribing treatments. In addition, he knows that typically his patient will be paying at least part of the cost of the services directly.

For the patient's part, it never enters his mind that his physician would prescribe treatments of dubious value in order to obtain some personal financial benefit or do anything less than follow the established ethical standards of the profession.

Clearly, this is a romanticized picture of a relationship, evoked from a time when the process of care was much less complex and when the potential benefit of medical care was much more limited than it is now. Nonetheless, contemporary patients tend to imagine something approximating such a relationship; in numerous studies patients tend to express dissatisfaction when certain of its key elements are missing. They complain when they feel the doctor showed a "lack of personal interest [and provided] insufficient explanation of their condition" (Freidson, 1970, p. 103). Moreover, although in some respects "the material on patient satisfaction is equivocal, . . . none contradicts the idea that emotional satisfaction on the part of the patient seems more likely to be gained from a physician who is in a position to be more immediately responsive to (and dependent on) the patient than are group physicians who have obligations to a work organization" (Freidson, 1970, p. 103).

We present this idealized picture of the physician-patient relationship for two main reasons.

First, although it appears to be what patients—and even many physicians (Heineke & Davidson, 1993)—would like, a number of features of modern American society have conspired to make it less and less likely that they will find it, at least not in its traditional form. As we saw in the previous chapter, this is partly because organizations now occupy a much larger part of the health care scene in this country than they used to, and many of them operate under financial constraints that tend to put a premium on the time a physician spends with a patient. Since many physicians in organizations keep relatively regular work schedules, a patient's personal physician may not be the clinician who sees him whenever he comes for care. Traditionally, when patients had a doctor who practiced alone and was always on call, he was the one who provided the service. Conversely, the availability of technology that was not present in the storied days of old may reduce the negative implications of this fact. In some organizations, automated information systems, to cite one example, create records that a covering physician can access when the regular doctor (who may not need them as much since he knows the patient) is unavailable. It is one of the tasks of management to make sure that those systems are in place and serving this need. The task may be easier to accomplish in a staff- or group-model HMO, or even in a hospital, than it is in an IPA, but the need is no less in any multiphysician group.

If the manager makes clinical information systems accessible and if clinicians learn to use them effectively, it may be possible to transfer a patient's loyalty and trust from the individual doctor to the organization. If so, then a sick patient can have the same confidence and no more anxiety when the regular physician is unavailable and another physician from the same organization is filling in. A covering physician with access to an electronic medical record can have most of the information—history, previous treatments, drug allergies, and other pertinent issues—needed to provide care that is more than episodic since it is based on knowledge of what went before and is connected to what will come later. This scenario contrasts favorably with the all-too-frequent alternative: a stranger appears in an emergency room or clinic with symptoms, a vague story of complaints, and no knowledge of prior test results.

The second reason we talk about doctors and patients in such a romanticized way is that although this portrait may seem to be a throwback to an earlier age when life was simpler and medical science was much less powerful, we show later (in Chapter Six) that *the absence of certain elements of the old doctor-patient relationship actually reduces the quality of patient care delivered* and undermines the viability of health care organizations by weakening the ties patients feel to them. As a result, we argue that an essential element of the job of health care managers is to *create conditions* under which it is once again *possible* for physicians to develop and sustain strong affective relationships with patients.[1] Managers must then *encourage* physicians to do just that. In addition, they must use modern information technology and other tools in a deliberate attempt to translate some of the patient's attachment to the physician into loyalty to the organization as well.

Ironically, some of those same characteristics of or opportunities represented by modern health care organizations contribute to what can be technically better care than was the norm in earlier times. Among these opportunities, as already noted, are regular work schedules, which reduce physician fatigue, and automated information systems, which reduce dependence on either a single individual physician (who is not always there) or on that physician's fallible memory. Conversely, these elements of the modern health care scene create important challenges which must be overcome if their large potential is to be realized. One such challenge is to find ways to reduce the scale of medical care to more human terms. Another is to develop reliable methods for sharing information between doctors so that the benefits of sophisticated equipment used to diagnose and treat patients are in fact achieved and not offset by poor communication. We return to this idea later.

Before we get to that part of the story, however, we lay some additional groundwork by discussing the changing health care system as it is experienced by its major players: the citizens and employers who purchase care and the physicians and health care managers who provide it. We begin, in the remainder of this chapter, by examining conditions that provide the context in which the relationship between patient and physician must develop. To a considerable extent, this is a discussion of obstacles that make it difficult to achieve the physician-patient relationship we have just described.

## The Mobility of the Population

In 1991–92, 17 percent of the population moved from one residence to another. Of those, 11 percent stayed in the same county and 6 percent moved to a different county, although half of the latter group stayed in the same state. Thus, at least 6 percent of the population in that one year moved to a location in which they would not be able to retain their primary physician (U.S. Bureau of the Census, 1994, p. 31). Moreover, between 17 percent and 20 percent mobility has occurred in each year since the late 1960s (Long, 1990, p. 48).

To obtain an estimate of unduplicated moves during the period, we consider several factors. First, some of those who moved did so more than once, especially because the age group that dominates the mobile population is young adults from twenty to twenty-nine, many of whom are looking for a rewarding job and/or a place to settle for the long term. Also, some of that mobility was probably situational—that is, a response to unstable economic conditions locally, if not nationally—and therefore not representative of a consistent pattern.

Nonetheless, it is reasonable to estimate that in the decade of the 1980s, 40 percent or more of the population moved far enough away from their previous residence that they were not able to maintain a personal relationship with a physician. (Physicians move, too, and their mobility also affects the stability of patient-physician relationships.) Further, from the National Health Interview Survey we learn that of the 34 percent who moved in each of three overlapping three-year intervals (1975–1978, 1976–1979, and 1977–1980), about half moved more than once in the period (Tucker & Urton, 1987, p. 266).

Regardless of the precise numbers, it is apparent that ours is a mobile society. With so many relationships being relatively recent, with no history, and perhaps unstable, the fabric of the society is much more loosely woven than in the past. In this context, health care is just one more impersonal element in an increasingly impersonal world. Thus, when they are sick and vulnerable, many people are putting their lives in the hands of strangers (Rothman, 1991).

In this context, one of the life tasks faced by people who are new to a community is to identify physicians who can care for them. The traditional method is word of mouth from neighbors or colleagues who tell the newcomer the name of their internist, pediatrician, or gynecologist. Some health care organizations are at an advantage in this scenario, since instead of looking for several convenient and congenial independent physicians a family may decide to select a single organization. Indeed, many HMOs create a user-friendly process for choosing physicians. They provide lists of available physicians by specialty, location, and hospital affiliation. Staff- or group-model HMOs, for which hospital affiliation is common to all physicians, may provide additional information (such as a physician's age, gender, medical school, and residency).

Even unattached individuals—often young, healthy, and not in immediate need of physicians—may choose an HMO because it tends to be easy to deal with and relatively inexpensive. The HMO offers a ready-made health care system, which they can access in the infrequent instances when they get sick instead of having to scramble during the illness to find a physician-stranger. Other people, for one reason or another, do nothing in advance of need for health care and then rely on still other organizations, typically hospital emergency departments or nearby storefront clinics, for infrequent episodic care.

## Paying for Care

For many Americans, especially young adults as we have just seen, one obstacle to long-term relationships with primary care physicians has been their mobility. Another has been variations in the ability to pay for care and, increasingly in contemporary times, the role of insurance. Yet, as commonplace as this observation appears to Americans in the 1990s, as recently as 1960 private health insurance paid for only 21 percent of all health expenditures. In contrast, 56 percent was paid directly out-of-pocket by ordinary patients and their families to doctors and other caregivers (Table 3.1).

In the period between 1960 and 1993, two major trends stand out.

First, by the latter year, those direct, out-of-pocket payments had fallen to only 20 percent of personal health expenditures, *a striking drop of 36 percentage points since 1960.*

Table 3.1. Personal Health Care Expenditures, by Source of Funds, Selected Years, 1960–1993.

| Year | Total | Out-of-Pocket Payments | Private Health Insurance | Other Private Funds | Governments | |
|---|---|---|---|---|---|---|
| | | | | | Federal | State & Local |
| Amount in Billions | | | | | | |
| 1960 | $23.9 | $13.3 | $5.0 | $0.4 | $2.1 | $3.0 |
| 1970 | 64.9 | 25.6 | 15.2 | 1.7 | 14.6 | 7.8 |
| 1980 | 220.1 | 61.3 | 64.1 | 7.7 | 63.4 | 23.6 |
| 1990 | 612.4 | 138.3 | 206.7 | 24.0 | 178.1 | 65.3 |
| 1993 | 782.5 | 157.5 | 258.0 | 30.0 | 259.0 | 78.1 |
| Per Capita Amount | | | | | | |
| 1960 | $126 | $70 | $26 | $2 | $11 | $16 |
| 1970 | 302 | 119 | 71 | 8 | 68 | 36 |
| 1980 | 936 | 261 | 273 | 33 | 270 | 100 |
| 1990 | 2,361 | 533 | 797 | 92 | 687 | 252 |
| 1993 | 2,920 | 588 | 963 | 112 | 966 | 291 |
| Percent Distribution | | | | | | |
| 1960 | 100.0 | 55.9 | 21.0 | 1.7 | 8.9 | 12.5 |
| 1970 | 100.0 | 39.1 | 23.6 | 2.5 | 22.7 | 12.0 |
| 1980 | 100.0 | 27.8 | 29.1 | 3.5 | 28.8 | 10.7 |
| 1990 | 100.0 | 22.6 | 33.8 | 3.9 | 29.1 | 10.7 |
| 1993 | 100.0 | 20.1 | 33.0 | 3.8 | 33.1 | 10.0 |

Source: Adapted from Levit et al., National Health Expenditures, 1993, *Health Care Financing Review*, 1994, p. 281.

Second, private and public third parties together accounted for 80 percent of personal health care expenditures in 1993. Private insurance increased by 12 percent to about one-third of the total. Federal spending, which had been less than 9 percent in 1960, zoomed to more than 33 percent by 1993. Thus the public-sector third-party share of the total doubled to 43 percent of all personal health care expenditures.

As a result of these trends, the inability to pay for care became a much less important deterrent to using services for most Americans, and demand for care grew. The prodigious growth in total expenditures was in fact fueled by this shift to third-party payment. With so much money available, providers—including even office-based private physicians—were less constrained both in setting prices, which rose dramatically, and in providing services. The large increases created pressures to limit spending; those pressures in turn contributed to the trend away from the traditional doctor-patient relationship.

## Employment and Health Insurance

Employers are important in this discussion because for most Americans they arrange and (in whole or in part) pay for health insurance for their employees, and in many cases for employees' families as well. In 1990, they covered 70 percent of the population under age sixty-five (Congressional Budget Office, 1991, p. 69). Half of the rest were uninsured.

Such a large share of total expenditures increasing at such a prodigious rate creates obvious problems for companies trying to earn a profit in competitive markets in a demanding global economy. Before examining the steps these organizations have taken to cope with this burden and their implications for physician-patient relationships, we need to note that a system of insurance based on employment also affects those citizens who either are not employed or who work for companies that do not provide coverage. The system of insurance also affects those people who are hired as part-time workers or on a contract basis so that companies can save money by *not* providing benefits.

One effect on those Americans without health insurance is that when they do use care, they often go not to individual physicians but to health care organizations—especially hospital emergency departments and other episodic caregivers—because they are more likely to be able to receive care without having to pay. Hospital emergency departments have ethical, if not legal, obligations to provide care in emergency or urgent situations whether or not patients can pay (Griffith, 1993, p. 19). Moreover, they must often provide at least some service to determine whether or not the patient has a true emergency. This is especially the case with children, who are less able to communicate what is wrong with them. Although it is impossible to overstate the enormous capabilities of physicians highly trained in emergency medicine and the well-equipped, technologically sophisticated hospital emergency departments in which they practice, it is also true that for the relatively routine treatment of common acute illnesses or injuries, which they are often called upon to provide, these are neither the best clinicians nor the most appropriate sites of care. They can do little more than treat the symptoms presented to them in the episode and they often are handicapped by the absence of relevant information (which might have been found in an ongoing patient record). Moreover, other physicians, even those working in the same emergency department, who provide the necessary follow-up care a few days later often do not even have a record of the ailment that brought the patient to the hospital originally. In other words, the technology, if harnessed, can result in improved service; but without deliberate action to make it happen, it will not serve that purpose.

Although many forces tend to weaken or disrupt the ties between individual patients and individual physicians, we should not lament the passage of a simpler era. Neither should we be confident that the full potential of the modern age will be realized unless we take the steps to make things so. We return to these themes later. In the meantime, we need to understand more about the contribution to these trends made by employers' efforts to contain their health insurance expenditures.

## Employers and the Cost of Health Care

In providing most of the private health insurance in the United States, as we have just seen, employers have been concerned for many years about growing costs. In spite of considerable effort, however, the strategies adopted to limit their financial exposure have not worked reliably except in isolated instances, or temporarily. In the next few pages, we identify these strategies and discuss the extent to which they, too, contribute to weakening the ties between individual patients and individual physicians and forcing both into organizational settings.

Trying to reduce their health care expenditures, employers have purchased lower-priced coverage for their employees, charged employees part of the premium cost, raised cost-sharing amounts, eliminated dependents from coverage, reduced covered services, and limited the choice of carrier or provider. That the issues raised by these strategies are important to employees is illustrated by the number of strikes in which the main focus has been health insurance benefits and at the end of which workers have given up pay increases to retain employer payment of health insurance premiums (Brailer & Van Horn, 1993, p. 128). Ironically, these measures, which clearly have not contained health care costs at the system level, often have failed even to bring individual employer costs under control.

In addition, companies have formed coalitions with other businesses to increase their purchasing power vis-à-vis insurers in local markets. That strategy often has two parts: providing information so that employers can act as more rational purchasers themselves; and in some cases, especially for small employers, attempting to pool risks and form larger purchasing groups in order to obtain better rates.

As we saw earlier, 70 percent of the population under sixty-five has private insurance, most of it provided by employers, who spend billions of dollars on it. For years, they have been expending considerable effort to contain those expenditures but have had limited success to date. A survey of public and private employers conducted by KPMG Peat Marwick and Wayne State University revealed that premiums increased an average of 8.5 percent between spring 1992 and spring 1993, "the lowest rate of increase in health insurance premiums and the first year of single-digit increases since 1986–1987" (Gabel, Liston, Jensen, & Marsteller, 1994, p. 328;

Gabel, DiCarlo, Sullivan, & Rice, 1990; Sullivan, Miller, Feldman, & Dowd, 1992). The increases were lower for large companies than for small ones and for conventional plans compared to managed care plans. Nonetheless, the rate of increase remained higher than the rate of inflation.

Not only was the annual rate of increase still higher than the rate of inflation, but expenditures were high to begin with. Across all plans, average monthly premiums in 1991 for individual coverage ranged from $143 to $188, and for family coverage from $349 to $543. Annualized, these monthly averages came to between $1,716 and $2,256 for individuals and between $4,188 and $6,516 for families (Gabel, Liston, Jensen, & Marsteller, 1994, p. 330). Rates tended to vary by size of employer (higher for smaller companies) and by type of plan (higher premiums tend to be associated with fewer restraints on utilization).

Moreover, health care costs as a percentage of total employee compensation have also been climbing. In 1985, 25 percent of employers reported that health care costs were less than 6 percent of total compensation; only 7 percent said the costs were 20 percent or more. By 1990, only five years later, the situation had reversed. Six percent of companies were in the lowest category, and 28 percent were spending 20 percent or more of employee compensation on health care benefits (Society for Human Resource Management, 1990, p. 7).

## What Employers Did to Contain Expenditures

### They Bought Less-Expensive Indemnity Policies

Stimulated in part by their desire to save on their expenditures for health care benefits and in part by the competitive actions of enterprising insurers, employers bought less-expensive conventional indemnity policies. This strategy may have started when commercial companies, sensing a lucrative market, began to offer experience-rated policies to employers with young, healthy workforces. Even though initially the policies were less expensive, this turned out to be an unsuccessful cost-containment strategy for several reasons. For one thing, some aggressive insurers who thought the biggest challenge was to get a toehold in the market quoted prices that were simply too low and had to be raised when the first contract expired. For another, except in very large groups utilization is inherently unstable, especially since physicians, hospitals, and others in a fee-for-service market have strong incentives to furnish services. The market for services is beyond the control of either a single insurer or a lone employer, neither of which can exert much influence (Enthoven & Kronick, 1989; Davidson, 1992).

Finally, even in an insurance market that *is* competitive, the reference price is the highest one, not the lowest. As part of a multifaceted strategy, insurers attempt to use price to attract business by charging less than their competitors. In setting their prices, however, they are constrained by their costs, since at a minimum they want prices to cover costs. But because they are not able to lower their costs indefinitely, they also cannot reduce their prices below those of their competitors indefinitely. If we assume that no insurer is able to cover everyone, the result is a market characterized by multiple companies offering policies over a relatively narrow range of prices, which are close enough that all can be viable. The price each insurer must beat, therefore, is the one at the top of that relatively narrow range. The result tends to be that insurers "shadow price" or "snuggle under" the price of that reference company (Foulkes, 1987). Given this scenario, it is not rational for insurance companies continually to underprice one another. Thus, even if employers want to purchase insurance primarily on the basis of price, the benefits from doing so are limited.

Many large employers self-insured and absorbed the financial risk themselves. By doing so, they hoped to retain for themselves the profit insurers otherwise earn from collecting and investing the premiums. Such firms usually hired a third-party administrator to

process claims, estimate plan costs actuarially, and conduct utilization review (Health Insurance Association of America, 1992; Sullivan, Miller, Feldman, & Dowd, 1992). While this strategy may
save employers some money in premium dollars, expenditures are
subject to the inherent instability of utilization described above.
Therefore, whether the employer actually saves money overall is
uncertain.

## They Imposed Costs on Employees

### Premiums

Although historically employers paid the entire premium for their
employees (and often their families as well), some companies sought
to limit their expenditures by sharing the premium cost with
employees. This has become a very sensitive issue, especially among
unionized employees who see the effort as an attempt of big business unilaterally to take away some of their hard-won benefits. That
view, coupled with the special anxiety about being exposed to the
financial cost of serious illness—feelings fuelled by almost-daily stories in newspapers and on television news programs about hard-
working families bankrupted by an unexpected catastrophic illness
or accident—has led to numerous well-publicized strikes in which
health benefits were a central issue. Cimini and Behrmann (1992,
p. 21) write that "Probably the most common and most contentious
issue . . . was dealing with rapidly increasing health insurance premiums that reflected rising health care costs." Brailer and Van Horn
(1993, p. 128) confirm that conclusion and quantify it, reporting
that "the percentage of strikes in which health benefits were a major
issue rose from 18 percent in 1986 to 78 percent in 1989 and is still
high. . . . [W]ell over 80 percent of strikes arise in large part from
health care concerns, and upwards of 90 percent are triggered by
companies shifting costs to employees."

Nonetheless, although 83 percent of full-time employees were
reported to have medical care coverage through their work in

1989–90, employers paid the full premium for less than half, 46 percent. Still fewer paid the full cost of family policies (Grossman, 1992, p. 37). Moreover, "employees contributed a greater share of the cost of premiums in 1993 than in 1988" for both conventional and HMO coverage. "For example, employees contributed 18.5 percent of the total cost for single conventional health coverage and 29 percent of the cost for family coverage in 1993—up from the 1988 averages of about 10 percent and 25 percent for individual and family coverage, respectively" (Gabel, Liston, Jensen, & Marsteller, 1994, p. 331).

## Cost-Sharing

Besides charging employees part of the premium cost, many employers also sought to impose costs on the actual utilization of services. In insurance, the concept of "moral hazard" means that, to the extent the event can be controlled, having insurance increases the probability that the risk being insured against will occur because a temptation exists to use the insurance (Koch, 1993, pp. 303–304). If health insurance increases the likelihood of utilization and therefore expenditures, then a reasonable strategy for controlling that utilization is to impose barriers to utilization without prohibiting it altogether. Following this thinking, employers have required employees to pay a part of the cost of the service directly.

Three primary devices are used to this end, each with different incentives. A *deductible* is the amount the employee must spend out of his or her own pocket before the insurance takes effect. If the deductible is $100, for example, then when the employee is sick early in the year he or she may hesitate longer before agreeing to spend $25 for an office visit (since the entire charge would need to be paid) than would happen later when the deductible has been met and the insurer will pay for the visit. Although a deductible may therefore deter utilization prior to its having been met, once an amount equal to the deductible has been spent, it has no further effect. Separate deductibles usually apply to each member of a family, although an annual family maximum is also common. Sometimes the annual deductible is divided in fourths and a separate amount (say, $25) is applied in each quarter of the benefit year. Gabel reports a wide range of actual deductibles, which varied considerably by plan type and firm size (Gabel, Liston, Jensen, & Marsteller, 1994, p. 332).

*Co-insurance* is a *percentage* applied to each claim, some to be paid by the insurer and the rest by the insured. The most common co-insurance is 80–20, with the employee being responsible for 20 percent of the cost of each bill.

*Co-payments* are *dollar amounts* to be paid by the employee with each use of a particular service. They tend to be rather small amounts and are applied most commonly to visits and prescriptions by HMOs, which usually have no other cost sharing, and by point-of-service plans. Cost sharing is often limited to an annual maximum out-of-pocket expenditure, commonly in the range of $500 to $2,000.

### Offering Multiple Plans

Originally, each employer offered a single plan, which covered all employees. In the search for less-expensive arrangements, many began to offer choices to their employees, sometimes with financial incentives for choosing the one thought to be the most effective at controlling excess utilization. A 1990 survey of 1,251 corporate members of the Society for Human Resource Management found that 57 percent of respondents offered a single plan, 21 percent offered two plans, and 22 percent offered three or more plans. It is worth noting that of those offering only a single plan, 38 percent were self-insured and only 5 percent and 12 percent respectively offered HMO or PPO coverage. Of the firms offering at least two plans, more than 60 percent offered HMOs, and more than 10 percent offered PPOs (Society for Human Resource Management, 1990, p. 6). Anecdotal evidence suggests that some large employers are dropping traditional indemnity plans or substantially increasing the price to their employees and adding restrictions. For example, for the 1993–94 benefit year, Boston University employees who wanted to continue in a traditional Blue Cross/Blue Shield indemnity plan were required to pay $255.29 per month for family coverage, but only $169.80 if they switched to a Blue Cross/Blue Shield IPA/POS plan.[2] Further, no employee who was not already covered by the indemnity plan was permitted to select it because it was being phased out. For 1994–95, employees no longer had the option of selecting an indemnity plan at all.

## Dropping Coverage

The ultimate imposition of dollar costs is for employers to drop coverage for their employees altogether. In this regard, two statistics are particularly noteworthy. First, "77 percent of employees worked in firms that offered health benefits in 1991. This figure declined from 81 percent in 1989" (Sullivan, Miller, Feldman, & Dowd, 1992, p. 173). Yet, although more than three-fourths of American *workers* still had employer-sponsored health benefits in 1991, only 40 percent of American *companies* with two or more workers offered coverage. "While nearly all large firms continued to offer health insurance, small firms showed a decrease in coverage" (Sullivan, Miller, Feldman, & Dowd, 1992, pp. 173–174).

Even though the percentage reductions in coverage are relatively small, the trends represented by these figures are disturbing for two reasons. One is simply that the percentages represent hundreds of thousands, if not millions, of individuals, who will suffer greatly if serious illness or accident strikes. The other is that newspaper accounts indicate these trends are continuing and may even be accelerating, resulting in still more Americans without coverage. Economic conditions are producing additional layoffs from large companies, new jobs are being created by start-up companies that cannot afford coverage for their employees, and federal and state governments have failed to protect citizens from the loss of their insurance (Freudenheim, 1995).

### They Imposed Nonmonetary Barriers to Utilization

#### Managed Care Arrangements

Employers entered into contracts with organizations—including HMOs, PPOs, and POS plans—that combined insurance with provider-imposed mechanisms for restricting utilization. In some cases, subscribers were required to select a primary care physician, whom they were to contact first whenever they needed service. That physician would provide the needed care directly, refer the patient to a more appropriate provider (for example, a subspecialist), or admit the patient to a hospital. In this case, the primary care physician would "manage" the patient's use of the health care system, thereby avoiding the use of unnecessary services that results when the patient manages his own care and seeks a specialist's services on his own. Although managed care imposes constraints on use of the health care system, it can be a relatively benign measure if the primary care physician and the patient come to know each other well enough that they can approximate the physician-patient relationship described previously.

Another method of managing care is to require prior authorization of the use of certain services. In this instance, the physician must contact a "case manager," describe the patient's condition, and request authorization to admit the patient to the hospital or to perform a certain procedure. Here, the decision maker is at the other end of a telephone line, a stranger to both the physician and the patient, asking a predetermined set of questions and approving or disapproving the request based on whether the answers fit an established protocol. This method of case management evokes great concern from physicians and patients alike about "cookbook medicine" and fails to take account of extenuating personal circumstances that may be important in a given situation.

Situated between these two forms is a method that makes use of a primary care physician as care manager but limits that physician's choices by identifying a set of approved providers, including physicians, laboratories, pharmacies, and others. Providers may be on the approved list because of their affiliation with the primary care physician's hospital and their agreement to accept discounted fees for services. The patient not only needs to be referred by the primary care physician but in some instances is also dependent on the latter's finding on the approved list a suitable cardiologist, for example, who is accessible in the clinically indicated length of time. While it may be appropriate for a patient to use a hospital emergency room in the aftermath of an accident, follow-up care must be provided or authorized by the primary care physician. Since the follow-up must often occur on the next day (changing dressings after treatment for second-degree burns, to take the example in the vignette "Paying the Bill" in Chapter One), the primary care physician may have difficulty finding an appropriate specialist on the approved list who has an open appointment on short notice.

### Mandatory Second Opinions

Some employers *required* employees to obtain second opinions when their physicians recommended surgery. The cost of the second opinion was covered by the insurance policy, and usually the plan would cover the surgery if the patient decided to go ahead with it notwithstanding a disagreement between two physicians' opinions. Some policies would permit a third opinion, as well. This device was introduced following evaluation of an innovation introduced in the 1970s by a large union's health plan in New York. Studies showed that surgery rates were reduced and that the savings more than covered the cost of the second opinions. In addition, no evidence was reported either that the lower rates reflected only delays in procedures or that patients' health suffered as a result of forgoing the surgery (McCarthy & Finkel, 1978; Grafe, McSherry, Finkel, & McCarthy, 1978).

### Prior Authorization

Another common device introduced in recent years has been the requirement that in order to be covered certain expensive services must be approved *in advance* by a representative of the insurer.

Typically, prior to hospitalization or surgery, a physician is required to call or submit a form to an insurance-company reviewer (often a nurse), who asks questions according to a protocol and, depending on the answers, approves the service or denies it. Usually the physician and patient have the right to appeal to a designated physician reviewer if they believe a denial was made in error.

A similar procedure is often followed *during* hospitalization, which typically either is approved for a specified number of days or is reviewed after a predetermined length of stay. At the review, a physician who believes a patient still needs hospital care must persuade the reviewer, who again refers to a protocol in making the decision. If additional days are denied, the physician may appeal; but if the insurer's final decision is that the stay is not necessary, a claim will be rejected.

## They Imposed Post-Utilization Conditions

Concurrent review of patient care gives the plan the opportunity to intervene to stop the delivery of services considered to be unnecessary. In that way, costs are avoided because resources are not used. As might be expected, however, physicians especially—and patients as well, particularly when physicians inform them of the process—resent the intrusion of a "clerk" on the telephone deciding whether a particular patient needs services and, if so, which services and how much. They complain that the reviewers cannot assess extenuating circumstances that make a specific patient's situation atypical. Moreover, the protocols are based on statistical probabilities derived from population studies, which always encompass a range of behaviors. Thus, even if the modal condition is adopted as the standard, a substantial proportion of patients will not fit the protocol. While aggregated clinical data may be a useful basis for developing practice *guidelines*, rigid application to individual patients of protocols based on statistics not only removes the human element from medicine but is an inappropriate use of the research in any case. Moreover, any unfortunate health consequences resulting from the failure to treat the patient would probably fall on the practitioner; it is unlikely that the insurer's refusal to pay for a service would absolve the clinician of liability for those results.

In view of these considerations, some plans review the care *after* it has been delivered instead of intervening during the medical care process. In the mid 1970s, the Medicare program tolerated, if it did not actually encourage, *retrospective denial* of payments to physicians and other providers who had already delivered the services for which they were submitting a bill. This mechanism is subject to many of the same criticisms as prior authorization, as well as the additional objection that it unfairly penalizes a presumably honest clinician who was providing a covered service which, based on professional judgment, was needed by the patient. Regardless of its outcome in any given case, a policy of retrospective denials is likely to have a dampening effect on the willingness of providers to treat patients covered by that plan.

If the goal is to influence *future* clinical decisions, that result can be achieved with fewer ill feelings by a plan that provides feedback to the physician to show that his *pattern* of care (not a decision for an individual patient) somehow departed from the norm. This device, *utilization review*, has also been applied for many years to utilization under Medicare, currently through peer review organizations (PROs) and predecessor organizations. For example, a physician who tended to order lab tests much more frequently than colleagues did—especially after patient complaint, diagnosis, and other characteristics were controlled statistically—might on his own rethink the extent to which he would order tests in the future. Perhaps he would recognize that he was using them as an unneeded crutch and reduce his ordering practices. In such an instance, the information could be provided privately, and the physician could change his practice patterns without having to expose his decisions to an argumentative reviewer in an adversarial environment. On the theory that a prime motivation of physicians is to serve their patients well, this outcome may be especially likely if the physician would suffer no financial loss as a result of using a higher threshold for ordering tests.

## They Have Formed or Joined Business Coalitions

The failure of all of these devices to control their health care costs adequately led some businesspeople to a different hypothesis of what the real problem was: that they were single employers acting alone. They did not have enough information about the variety of insurers or providers to make truly informed decisions as to the value of the coverage and price being offered. Additionally, they were not responsible for enough business to be able to influence either a large insurer or a provider of services. If they pooled their resources and the lives they covered with those of other employers in the community, perhaps they would be in a stronger position both to acquire the information they needed to act as rational consumers of coverage and to negotiate effectively with insurers and providers. This kind of thinking led to the formation of business coalitions in large markets throughout the country.

Many have not proceeded beyond the point of holding meetings in which participants discuss their problems and share their latest ideas for solving them, or of collecting and providing information to member organizations. In some of the latter cases, moreover, the coalitions have limited data and have not been able to analyze it in ways that have proven useful to members.

Some coalitions, however, have begun to act as purchasers for small or medium-sized businesses in their markets. Although published reports contain claims of reduced prices or other savings, the financial results have tended to be limited and/or transitory and have not been subjected to scrutiny by independent researchers. Nonetheless, this concept has appeal in a competitive environment and is a major component of the "managed competition" strategy (Enthoven, 1993; Ellwood, Enthoven, & Etheredge, 1992; Enthoven & Kronick, 1989).

## Conclusions

The failure to control health care expenditures, despite years of trying, has led many companies to want to get out of the business of providing health care coverage to their employees. Indeed, fewer than half of American companies do provide health insurance coverage (Sullivan, Miller, Feldman, and Dowd, 1992, p. 174). And for those which do still offer it, health insurance is an intransigent mystery: they do not understand it and cannot seem to do anything about it. The attempt to master health insurance is an expensive diversion from their main activities, and they have neither the expertise nor the capital to be effective at it. The familiar array of cost containment strategies described in this chapter has not stopped the financial hemorrhaging, and employer efforts in this regard have damaged their relations with employees. They have undercut employee loyalty to the companies; in the case of unionized workforces the result frequently has been costly strikes.

This failure to control health care expenditures leads us to two conclusions.

First, the smallest unit with the power to affect health insurance costs reliably without compromising the access of individuals to the services they need is the metropolitan market as a whole. The best that individual companies, even very large ones, can do is to control their own costs and influence the delivery of services to their own employees. Small or medium-sized companies cannot do even that; moreover, in part they must pay higher prices to help insurers and providers compensate for the tough bargaining with the large companies. Reasonable observers may differ as to whether successful actions at the level of a metropolitan market can be accomplished without government intervention and, if not, what the nature of that intervention should be.

Our second conclusion is that even where market-level reforms do succeed in holding the line on health insurance premiums, determined and sustained attention must be given to the actual delivery of services. If not, those insurance premiums will again begin to rise faster than inflation. More importantly, unless patients are treated in a timely manner with appropriate services delivered with skill, money will be wasted and individuals will be hurt. Some of the stories in Chapter One imply considerable room for progress on that score; examples later in this book reinforce the point.

It is not enough to pay an HMO a fixed capitation amount and relax. While that HMO has an incentive to limit its costs in delivering services, it can accomplish that goal in several ways. It can engage good doctors and other clinicians, create a culture committed to efficient and effective service to patients, and install operational systems that support that goal. Alternatively, it can erect barriers that make it difficult for patients seeking services to receive them. The bottom line is that the choices and actions the HMO and its clinicians take *after* the capitation rate is negotiated and the insurance contract is signed matter a lot.

Everyone in the role of patient (the individual employer, the family member, the provider of services) expects his own clinician's primary motivation to be to treat him well with the services he needs. Indeed, a large body of writing about the ethical basis of contemporary medical care, which has incorporated adaptations to the new conditions described earlier (prepayment, competition, the growing importance of technology), reaffirms the physician's historic commitment to his patients as the core idea (Jonsen, 1990; Veatch, 1977; and Griffith, 1993). Moreover, far from being a peripheral curiosity, these concepts are central to the success of medical care in the future. Today, however, the ethical provider is not a solitary physician but a complex health care organization operating under constraints that daily test their commitment to patients.

The trends identified here have caused many patients to lose confidence in the medical care system. Since today's services tend to be delivered under the auspices of health care organizations by their employees or contractors, one task of the managers of those organizations is to help restore that confidence.

## Effects on Relations Between Individual Patients and Physicians

The activities described in this chapter to contain health care costs have contributed to the growing tension in relations between patients and their physicians. Medical care no longer begins with a phone call from a patient to his or her personal physician in a small office nearby. Money and payment arrangements often intrude, and sometimes, as we have seen, other people become involved as well.

When new patients call a physician's office for an appointment, often one of the first questions they are asked concerns the anticipated method of payment. If the patient cannot demonstrate a high likelihood that he can pay (whether through insurance or otherwise), he may be denied an appointment. Moreover, some physicians refuse to deal with certain payers altogether. This practice, which at first was limited to the large public programs Medicare and Medicaid (Physician Payment Review Commission, 1990; Davidson, 1982), has spread to some of the private HMOs. It may take the form of saying that the physician is not accepting any more patients from Plan X or of offering an appointment so far in the future that the patient refuses to wait. Many physicians now take credit cards; although that may increase the probability of being paid, it also increases the extent to which the delivery of medical care resembles just another impersonal commercial transaction.

In addition to payment issues, tensions also arise from the fact noted earlier that some clinical decisions are made not in a private interaction between a patient and physician but with the involvement of a reviewer or clerk at an 800 number, perhaps in another part of the country. This is especially likely to be the case for those services that require prior authorization or for hospitalization in which the treating physician would like the patient to remain longer than the stay originally approved.

For individuals, another dimension of what can fairly be described as a deteriorating situation is the substantial anxiety many have about either losing their coverage or not having enough coverage for the services they will need (Blendon et al., 1993). The newspapers and other media are full of stories about hard-working, middle-class families who thought they had "good" coverage until some unexpected tragedy hit (Lewis, 1995), or families with a chronically ill child requiring continuing treatment, whose premiums—but not those of other members of their group—were raised so much that they could no longer afford to keep the coverage. Since such action by an insurer violates the risk-pooling principle that is fundamental to insurance, it is hard to avoid being both anxious and cynical.

Physicians harbor increasing resentment about intrusions on their medical judgment. They are the professionals with both the expertise and the responsibility to provide medical services to people who need them. Yet everywhere they turn, organizations interfere. Some establish arbitrary rules for receiving payment, so physicians "fudge" the claims they submit in order to obtain the payment to which they believe they are entitled. They learn how to write orders or requests for authorization that will be approved. They have a growing feeling that medical care has become a sick competition between them and "accountants" who make clinical decisions. Surveys show that many physicians claim they would not recommend medicine as a career for their own children or would not have entered it themselves if they had known how conditions would change after they entered practice (Altman, with Rosenthal, 1990). Many have the feeling that anonymous clerks at peer review organizations are scrutinizing their practice decisions, hoping to catch them in an error, and they have even become wary of their patients in an environment in which the threat of malpractice claims and suits has become a major preoccupation.

All of these events, many of which derive from employer efforts to contain health insurance costs, exemplify the growing prominence of organizations in the health care system and the deterioration in physician-patient relationships. They result from a series of individual decisions each of which may seem reasonable in itself, but which together add up to an increasingly dysfunctional health care system. Since organizations play an ever greater role, their performance is the key to creating a system that functions smoothly in taking effective care of patients, satisfies both patients and clinicians, is efficient, and in the process restores public confidence in American medicine. Although the challenge must be joined in organizations, these same health care organizations that absorb patients and physicians are themselves the source of much of the anxiety and the targets of much of the anger of physicians and patients alike.

It is in this environment that managers must function as the organizations' custodians. In order to attract clients, they need to attract physicians. In order to retain both, they need to create conditions inside the organizations that allow, and even encourage, physicians to build strong relationships with their patients, and which facilitate the smooth integration of responsive, high quality care gratifying to both groups. Indeed, we believe that one of the major challenges for health care organizations in the future is to restore the human scale and reintroduce the human dimension to medical care in the United States. It is the manager—the CEO, COO, medical director, a subordinate—who must ensure that the organization's goal of timely, responsive, effective, and efficient service to patients is achieved. But physicians and other clinical professionals provide the actual services, so managers accomplish these goals indirectly, by influencing physicians' clinical decisions.

These tasks would be difficult under any circumstances; they are made inordinately harder by the conditions described in this chapter. They are further complicated by the training, experience, and expectations of the physicians and managers on whose shoulders the challenges fall and to which we turn next.

# 4

. . . . . . . . . . . . . . . . . . . . . . . . . . . . . . . .

# Physicians and Managers
## The Search for Common Ground

Managers are responsible for the viability of contemporary health care organizations. Doctors are responsible for the organizations' clinical services. To a considerable extent, therefore, the interests of both groups of professionals are intimately connected to those of the organizations. Yet as we intimated in previous pages, the relationships between managers and doctors are often strained.

This is the case even though both groups have good reason to want their organizations to succeed and thereby have a common stake in organizational success. Both have an interest in attracting and serving large numbers of patients (at least up to a manageable limit). And to the extent that patients' choices of provider depend on their experience with the care they receive, both have an interest in effective delivery of good care to patients.[1]

Despite these common elements, the interests of these two groups are not identical. In addition to concern for the organization, they both also have personal and/or professional goals that are not the same even though they do overlap. For one thing, although both want to earn good incomes, the pay of one may depend on the other. Managers negotiate the financial arrangements with physicians, and although they want physicians to remain loyal to the organization and therefore be content, they also want to keep the organizations' costs (including pay to physicians) under control. By some measures, then, managers gain by constraining physician gains. Further, managers and physicians have different orientations to their work, growing out of their socialization through dissimilar education and professional associations.

In this chapter, we explore the similarities and differences among managers and physicians; we focus particularly on the impact that health care system trends have had on their relationships with one another. Here, we emphasize the sources of the strain between them. Later in this book, we seek means for breaking down some of the barriers to the achievement of their common goal of serving patients.

## Physicians

Physicians as a group have changed considerably in the last thirty years, and those changes have helped to shape the new health care system. At the same time, some of the changes we have already discussed have had an impact on physicians. In the first part of this chapter we discuss (1) how the physician group has changed; (2) behavioral responses of individual physicians to those changes, especially the fact that so many now have formal relationships with organizations; and (3) their attitudes toward these changes, and the contributions of their attitudes, work characteristics, and psychology to the prospects for improving the delivery of care in organizations. In the second half of the chapter, we take a comparable look at managers.

### Trends in the Numbers and Characteristics of Physicians

For many years, the number of doctors has increased faster than the population. From 1965 through 1992, the actual number of patient care physicians in the United States more than doubled while the population increased by only 30 percent (Roback, Randolph, & Seidman, 1993). To put it another way, in 1992, 77 additional physicians were available for every 100,000 Americans than was the case in 1965 (Table 4.1).

Table 4.1.  Patient Care Physicians and
Physician/Population Ratios, 1965–1992.

| Year | Number of Patient Care Physicians | Patient Care Physicians per 100,000 People | Population per Patient Care Physician |
|------|-----------------------------------|--------------------------------------------|--------------------------------------|
| 1965 | 259,418 | 132 | 760 |
| 1970 | 278,535 | 134 | 747 |
| 1975 | 311,937 | 142 | 703 |
| 1980 | 376,512 | 163 | 614 |
| 1985 | 448,820 | 185 | 541 |
| 1990 | 503,870 | 200 | 500 |
| 1992 | 535,220 | 209 | 479 |
| Change | +275,802 | +77 | −281 |
|  | (+106 percent) | per 100,000 | per M.D. |

Source: Adapted from Roback, Randolph, & Seidman, 1993.

Even if nothing else were going on, this growth in the numbers
of physicians would result in more competition among them. The
reason is elementary economics: to the extent that their work
derives from the health care needs of the population, which in a sta-
ble, developed society do not change much from year to year, each
physician will have less work than previously.[2]

The physician group has been changing along other important
dimensions as well, notably the dramatic growth in the number of
women in the field. In 1969–70, only 948 women enrolled as first-
year students in U.S. medical schools, accounting for 9.1 percent of
the entering class. By 1985–86, the number had grown to 5,800, or
34.2 percent (Bowman & Gross, 1986).

The specialty distribution is also important. In 1970, of 334,000
active physicians, 35 percent practiced in the primary care specialties of general or family practice, internal medicine, and pediatrics.
In 1992, although the absolute numbers of practicing physicians had
more than doubled, the proportion in primary care was exactly the
same (Roback, Randolph, & Seidman, 1993). This distribution of

generalists and specialists, which is almost the reverse of that in other developed countries (Schroeder, 1992), has important implications for the future of the U.S. system and for relations between physicians and managers in health care organizations. We return to this issue later.

## Responses to the Number of Physicians and Other Trends

To protect themselves from the consequences of such trends, doctors have done a number of things worth mentioning.

1.    They have increased the amount of care provided (Swedlow, Johnson, Smithline, & Milstein, 1992; Relman, 1992). In a fee-for-service system, offering more services translates into higher income; indeed, visit rates per physician have been increasing.

2.    More have become specialists, as we have already seen. While many cite the intellectual challenge of treating people with relatively uncommon conditions, the fact that specialists earn higher incomes than generalists is undoubtedly a factor as well (Roback, Randolph, & Seidman, 1993; Pope & Schneider, 1992).

3.    Related to the first two points is the fact that many specialists have provided general care to their specialty patients. McDermott described this phenomenon in the early 1970s, calling it "the hidden system of general care" (McDermott, 1974). He noted that patients who were referred to a cardiologist to be treated for a specific heart ailment, for example, often returned to that subspecialist later when unrelated problems arose. The subspecialist often obliged by providing general medical care, doing so in part in order to avoid losing the patient; but it is also important to note that the physician had the free time to do so: even in the 1970s, when McDermott was writing, we had more specialists than the medical conditions of the population apparently required.

While these last two strategies may have helped physicians cope with new market conditions for a time, fee-for-service medicine itself is under siege. New methods of payment place a premium on productivity; they encourage provision of the maximum reasonable amount of services for a given level of input.

Moreover, there is some evidence that private primary care physicians are coping with the new conditions *they* face by holding on to their patients longer before referring them to specialists. This tactic is a recognition that "physicians who refer to specialists often end up losing patients" (Asinof, 1990, p. A1). The *Wall Street Journal* reported on a study that "found some 37 percent of family and general practitioners lost patients because of referrals in the last year, with the average loss eight patients per doctor" (Asinof, 1990, p. A1).

4. Physicians have joined organizations, as noted in Chapter Two. Older practitioners especially have feared loss of patients and/or reduction of income, and they have complained that their decision making was increasingly constrained by insurers, the government, and employers. Some have joined organizations such as HMOs or hospitals to avoid losing patients and/or to protect most of their income. In making the move, they may even have been willing to give up some income in exchange for increased financial security.

Younger physicians have also joined organizations in large numbers. They often have entered practice with large debts from an expensive medical education that was probably privately financed. In a competitive market, debt-laden young physicians are attracted to organizations, which require no significant capital investment, pay salaries and malpractice premiums, and generate a clientele. As a result, they need not be concerned about building a practice or about having enough income to cover practice costs, achieve their desired lifestyle, and repay debts. The trade-off is that the potential salary at the peak of their careers may not reach what some doctors have made in private, fee-for-service practice over the last thirty years (that is, since the proliferation of private insurance and the introduction of Medicare and Medicaid).

Another reason young physicians join organizations is to have a more appealing lifestyle (which is to say, regular hours among other things). This is especially, though not exclusively, true for the growing number of female physicians, many of whom also want to have families.

A further reason is that professional practice in organizations can be more rewarding in nonfinancial ways as a result of opportunities for interaction with other professionals. Some physicians feel less isolated as members of an organization than as solo practitioners or as part of a small, single-specialty group.

As the last few paragraphs imply, not all doctors are alike. Nor do they respond identically to the changes occurring in the American health care system. It is not accurate to speak of "doctors" as if they are one undifferentiated group with common interests. As indicated, generational differences among physicians may be as important as professional similarities. Other important dimensions of difference are gender and whether the physicians are specialists or generalists, independent practitioners or members of a group, contractors or employees.

## Physician Attitudes Regarding the Changes

While the kinds of reality factors we have been discussing may lead physicians to diverge from the traditional pattern of solo, office-based practice ("More Doctors," 1986), it is not necessarily the case that they *enjoy* these new arrangements. Indeed, growing evidence suggests that many physicians are considerably discontented. Lewis and his colleagues found in a survey of internists that while more than 80 percent of respondents were satisfied with their relationships with patients, professional challenges, and interaction with colleagues, about half were *dis*satisfied with their current and potential income, and 60 to 70 percent were dissatisfied with the time they had for nonmedical interests and with their level of personal control over their own practice (Lewis, Prout, Chalmers, & Leake, 1991). Many physicians apparently feel they do not determine their own professional activities and that they work longer and harder for less income and a less certain future.

A *New York Times* report of a Gallup poll of physicians found that "almost 40 percent of the doctors interviewed said that based on what they now knew about medicine as a career, they would definitely or probably not enter medical school if they had a career choice to make again" (Altman, with Rosenthal, 1990, p. 1).

Anecdotal reports indicate that for many physicians, "hassles and red tape" from organizations reduce their satisfaction with medical practice (Steptoe, 1987, p. A1).

Other survey results reveal a mixed picture. In Dane County (Madison), Wisconsin, 69 percent of primary care physicians in group and employed practices were satisfied or very satisfied with their work situation. Differences among specialties were not statistically significant. "Physicians in the IPA who have had to change the most reported less clinical autonomy than those not in an HMO, but in all other respects . . . they were at least as, or more, satisfied . . . [as] those not in an HMO" (Schulz, Girard, & Scheckler, 1992, p. 303).

In a more recent national survey, high levels of satisfaction with practice—even under managed care arrangements—were again found, but the results were not uniform. For example, "managed care exerts its strongest negative influence on the levels of perceived autonomy in the areas of time management and patient selection" (Baker & Cantor, 1993, p. 262). The authors go on to say that "striking" differences were recorded among physicians who were asked whether they had the freedom to control their own work schedule. "Thirty-nine percent of HMO physicians, compared with 64 percent of employees of other employers and 82 percent of self-employed physicians, felt free to control their schedules. Among HMO physicians, specialists felt more autonomy, but 53 percent still felt that they did not have the freedom to control their own schedule" (Baker & Cantor, 1993, p. 262). Yet in other aspects of their work, including the ability to hospitalize their patients and to order tests and procedures, HMO physicians were no less, and in some cases more, likely to be satisfied than physicians in other settings.

From this picture, based more on newspaper accounts than systematic studies, we believe it is fair to say that many, but not all, physicians are having difficulty with the increasing prominence of organizational arrangements in medical care. Differences can be observed with regard to medical specialty, type of organizational setting, and the particular aspect of work or patient care being considered. Clearly, more needs to be learned through careful studies using a variety of methods.

## Implications for Managers

We noted earlier that managers are custodians of health care organizations. In that capacity, they have considerable responsibility regarding physicians and the work they perform. We make the assumption—one that not everyone shares, as we note in Chapter Six—that if they take "appropriate" measures (which we cannot yet define), they can positively affect physician behavior and attitudes about their work. In planning their strategies, managers should take note of certain generalizations about physician attributes, including training, socialization, and even psychological characteristics. Kurtz (1993) drew attention to these attributes in a paper in which he contrasted clinicians with managers. Bettner and Collins (1987) made a similar comparison that we have reproduced as Table 4.2.

We present these views because they reflect a widely held belief that characteristic attributes of individuals in the two groups account for much of the conflict between managers and doctors. It is important to point out that although these are plausible tendencies, they apparently derive from the authors' "general knowledge" and not from systematic research. The intragroup differences among physicians already noted in their reasons for joining organizations, attitudes about aspects of managed care, and other factors suggest that such generalizations are risky and should be viewed with caution until they are verified empirically.

Conversely, certain other characteristics of physicians can be accepted with more confidence. One is that medicine is a "consulting profession," which means that in contrast to "learned scientific professions" its members "survive by providing a varied lay clientele services that are expected to solve practical problems"

Table 4.2. Contrasting Characteristics of Managers and Physicians.

| Managers | Physicians |
| --- | --- |
| 1. They are hired as general managers. | They are entrepreneurial capitalists. |
| 2. They are multidisciplined. | They are specialists. |
| 3. They must control individuals. | They resist being controlled. |
| 4. They must establish rules of conduct. | They resist rules. |
| 5. They must serve many interests concurrently. | They are oriented to one group (patients). |
| 6. Their decisions are determined by policy (consensus). | They must make their own decisions. |
| 7. They view hospital cost control as a high priority. | They view hospital cost control as restrictive. |
| 8. They are realists. | They are idealists. |
| 9. They represent organizations. | They represent themselves. |

*Source:* Reprinted with permission from Bettner, M., & Collins, F. (1987). Physicians and administrators: Inducing collaboration. *Hospital and Health Services Administration, 32*(2), p. 154.

(Freidson, 1970, p. 22). An important implication of this observation is that physicians must be able to attract patients on the basis of patient beliefs about the value they will receive from the encounter. Thus, as noted earlier, physicians and managers share an interest in satisfying the "customer."

Second, modern physicians are presumed to have an array of services that reliably provide benefit to patients. That reliability is grounded in science, which in turn confers on physicians a legitimate claim to the license a state grants them to practice in ways that others cannot. Thus, they have a state-sanctioned "monopoly over the exercise of . . . [their] work" (Freidson, 1970, p. 88).

Third, individual physicians learn the knowledge, skills, attitudes, and ethical commitments they need in medical school and through supervised practical experience in hospitals (and increasingly in other clinical settings). The education and socialization the physician acquires during the training process are important "source[s] of much of his performance as a practitioner" (Freidson, 1970, p. 88).

But, fourth, physicians are also influenced by the settings in which they work. In fact, Freidson argues that "education is a less important variable than work environment" as a determinant of a physician's professional behavior (Freidson, 1970, p. 89). If he is right, then the manager of a health care organization has considerable opportunity to influence physician actions to serve their common interest in the organization's patients.

On this optimistic note, we continue this discussion with a brief examination of managers in the health care system.

## Health Care Managers

Managers of modern health care organizations have a difficult job indeed. Not only does the environment swirling around them make planning a guessing game to some degree, but they must also deal with a variety of groups, each of which is suffering considerable anxiety about what the future holds for its members.

In this section, we briefly describe the role health care managers enjoyed until the turbulence began to intensify in the last fifteen years. Then we identify key components of their job—both inside and outside the organization—and introduce the suggestion that their background, training, and experience have not prepared them particularly well to handle these challenges effectively. Before concluding, we attempt to connect the difficulties physicians face with the actions managers may take.

### The Old-Time Health Care Manager

Until recently, the field in which managers of health care organizations practiced was called "hospital administration," and for good reason. Hospitals indeed constituted the majority of health care organizations. The manager's tasks were thought of largely as acquiring the resources (that is, space, equipment, supplies, ancillary staff) physicians wanted, and arranging them so that the physicians' hospitalized patients could be cared for.

It should be recalled, as we saw in Chapter Two, that the original hospitals were little more than almshouses for the poor who were sick and had no family to care for them. Most medical care, such as it was, was provided by independent practitioners, often in the homes of their sick patients. It was not until the 1890s that hospitals began to transform themselves into institutions with the capacity to provide beneficial medical and surgical treatments. Control of hospitals, originally in the hands of lay boards and superintendents, passed to physicians because of the expertise that increasingly separated them from laypeople and because the facilities' fiscal health depended on the extent to which physicians brought in patients for care. As Rothman (1993, p. 19) notes, "When the process was completed, the lay people really had little to do except take care of the housekeeping and raise funds for new pavilions and equipment." With the explosion of private and public third-party payment beginning in the 1960s, even the laypersons' role as fund-raisers diminished. Hospitals were able to borrow funds for capital investment, at least to supplement charitable contributions, because they could use the vast sums they were earning from the provision of services to repay the loans.

The conceptualization of the hospital as "the doctor's workshop" conveys much of the thinking of this era of physician dominance. The administrator's job was to see to it that expert doctors had what they required for the care of their patients, who were hospitalized because they were presumed to be very sick. There were two effects that are relevant to our concerns. One is that the administrator's job depended on physicians. Doctors made known their "needs," and the administrator tried to fill them. To meet those needs, the administrator may have had to raise money, negotiate with suppliers, arrange for construction of new facilities, and accomplish other tasks, which required an understanding of finance, bargaining, and other skills. Although boards "frequently fought [with physicians] over escalating costs" (Rothman, 1993, p. 19), the amount of conflict was limited because in an era of cost-based reimbursement, lenders were plentiful and the need to raise money was not much of a constraint.

A second and related effect of the old system on managers was that they did not gain experience negotiating with physicians. Indeed, the issues they did discuss with physicians were often medical or scientific and technical, and therefore beyond their ken. Administrators tended to avoid discussion of those subjects as much as possible; when occasionally such topics came up anyway, they quickly found themselves in over their heads, no match for the expert physicians. Although administrators had an important role in the hospital and could take pride in their professional accomplishments, they were clearly secondary to physicians. Indeed, many hospitals institutionalized this relationship by insisting that the hospital's chief executive be a physician. If a professional hospital administrator was hired, he would become the chief operating officer—reporting to the physician chief executive.

As a result, prior professional experience did not prepare administrators either to lead the army of health care organizations that dot the modern landscape or to assume the new, more complex management roles that changing conditions have thrust upon them. Confronting the challenges of rapid systemic change, which would be daunting under any circumstances, health care managers as a group have thus been disadvantaged by experience that prepared them poorly to deal with those tasks.

Nor does it appear that they were adequately prepared by formal professional training in health administration programs, which tend to emphasize finance, accounting, and other "business" skills. Process skills, such as leadership and methods for influencing behavior in organizations, received limited attention, sometimes being denigrated as "soft" in comparison to the more quantitative and (some would therefore say) more "real" fiscal element.

## Tasks of the Contemporary Health Care Manager

The tasks of contemporary health care managers vary in detail by type of organization. Hospitals, which provide secondary and tertiary care, engage in different activities than managed care organizations (MCOs), which emphasize primary care and other ambulatory services. The common denominator is the organizational interest in the delivery of quality services in a responsive yet efficient manner.

Nonetheless, the increasing importance of financial constraints places growing demands on managers as custodians of all of these care-providing organizations. These constraints may be embodied in methods of payment, such as Medicare's prospective payment system for hospital services or capitation payment for comprehensive HMO services, or they may derive from reduced demand for inpatient hospital services (and the accompanying need to adapt by diversifying, by forming joint ventures with physicians, or by vertical integration with other providers). Whatever the source, the constraints give managers a powerful reason to be concerned about actual delivery of services, including the personnel and the processes that produce them. They cannot afford to be indifferent to clinicians' decisions about what care should be provided, who should provide it, where it should be offered, and with what equipment and supplies. If they are to be effective custodians of health care organizations, managers must concern themselves with those decisions and processes. Although the higher stakes for their organizations also give managers potentially more clout or leverage with physicians, they need to exercise that power judiciously. Undoubtedly some methods of attempting to influence physicians will be more successful in accomplishing their goals than others. We return to this issue later.

From anecdotal evidence, it appears that managers are particularly likely to focus on the cost of care. In contrast to quality, for example, cost is an issue that lends itself to easy measurement: how many dollars are being spent compared to the amount of income being brought in. Moreover, cost appears to be a "business" issue with which managers have greater standing or legitimacy than physicians, even though, since cost and quality are closely linked, managers must often address elements of the delivery of clinical services in order to deal with the cost issue.

Even in addressing the cost question, however, managers face a fundamental dilemma. To what extent should they either impose "rational" policies on the organization or engage clinicians in processes to solve problems raised by management? Regarding the cost of care, an example of the first approach is to determine that physicians are not "productive" enough, decide the problem is the absence of incentives for them to be so (that is, they are paid salaries that are independent of the number of patients they see), and hire consultants to design incentive compensation schemes that are intended to increase productivity. But if physicians are unhappy with the new payment arrangements, complaining they are overworked and underpaid, then unilateral imposition of those incentives may produce unwanted side effects without increasing productivity.

An alternative is for managers to define the problem more generally as the high cost of the care being delivered (that is, the cost per subscriber is higher than can be sustained in a competitive market and it is growing) and to engage clinicians in a process to describe it more precisely, identify its causes, and propose solutions. The latter might involve new work arrangements, including changes in compensation arrangements; but it might also include refinements in the care delivery processes, such as innovations that make it possible to reduce use of the "urgent care" clinic and/or out-of-plan use.

In what follows, we use the example of a staff-model HMO to illustrate some of the tasks and some of the choices managers face, particularly regarding the delivery of clinical services. Specific tasks and choices faced by managers in other types of health care organizations would be somewhat different.

At least two factors limit what the manager in any health care organization can do. First, the physicians are professionals and thus presumably view the provision of beneficial service to patients as a first-order goal. In addition, they make decisions on the basis of their knowledge and experience, to a great extent answering to professional physician-colleagues as well as to the health care organization's managers (Freidson, 1970). Second, the organization—through its clinical staff—offers to the public professional services which by definition are not uniform or routine, and that often require the exercise of a considerable amount of judgment. These services are not off-the-shelf, like many products; instead, each one is "custom designed" for the particular patient.

For both these reasons—as well as because of modern theories of management (Deming, 1986)—managers cannot order or instruct physicians how to take care of patients. Conversely, although they need to be somewhat less direct in their approach, they cannot afford to fail in their attempts to affect clinical practice. Seen in this light, their task is to influence, persuade, or encourage physicians to include the cost of services in their clinical calculus.

The organization may be assisted in this effort by hiring senior managers who are themselves experienced clinicians, who speak the same language as the HMO's practicing physicians, whose opinions will thus carry the weight of their own professional authority, and who—if the need should arise—can argue the merits of a particular clinical issue. Conversely, there is some evidence to indicate that HMO clinicians tend to view physicians who become managers more as managers than as physician colleagues (Heineke & Davidson, 1993). If this finding is generalized, it would tend to reduce the benefit to be gained by appointing physicians as managers. Regardless, in many cases it is not possible to hire physicians for these management roles.

The managerial functions of an HMO that relate to the delivery of its clinical services are numerous and varied.

### Recruitment of Physicians

This is a critical function in the life of an HMO, because if the "right" physicians are hired to begin with, many potential problems may be avoided. Issues to consider are the physicians' training and recommendations of teachers or chiefs of service; their commitment to what might be called "a conservative style" of practice; and their prior knowledge of HMOs and prepayment. Physicians are interested in working in HMOs for a variety of reasons, some more compatible with the organization's twin goals (effective service, delivered efficiently) than others. With the high cost and extended period of medical training these days, for example, some relatively new doctors may find the steady income and security of a staff-model HMO appealing for the short run but want to leave after a few years for a more traditional fee-for-service practice or another type of MCO. These physicians may give only minimal attention to the importance of cost controls, which they consider to be primarily for the benefit of the organization. Others may believe that the prepayment concept is quite sensible: on the one hand, in making clinical decisions physicians do not need to be concerned about putting extra financial burdens on their patients; on the other hand, they need not feel they have to do more for the patient than is really necessary in order to produce additional income, as some may be tempted to do in the fee-for-service mode.

The point is that selection of physicians who are "good" for prepaid practice is not just a matter of choosing between individuals with the best clinical credentials (unless the meaning of clinical credentials is broadened to include an effective understanding of the cost implications of clinical decisions). As a Pakistani physician studying in the United States told us, he believes his colleagues in Karachi have a better appreciation than American physicians of the actual value of the resources it takes to produce medical service because they practice in an environment of scarcity. Although an American HMO may not be as resource-poor as a health care facility in Pakistan, its managers are acutely aware that spendable resources are limited by the amount of premium revenue, and clinical decisions must be made with that simple fact in mind.

## Orientation of Physicians

Orientation to both the HMO concept and the particular HMO is another function performed by HMO managers. By definition, the HMO concept means a commitment to what is often called a conservative style of practice, one that orders tests and procedures when there is a clear expectation they will produce valuable benefits in diagnosis or treatment but forgoes them when indications are that their utility is marginal. It is a style that includes the cost of a service as one element in the informal calculation leading to the decision to provide a service—not the only consideration, to be sure, and not even the most important one, but legitimate nonetheless. It is a style that favors taking a more thorough history from the patient and conducting a more careful physical exam, but ordering fewer mechanical tests and performing fewer procedures.

Paradoxically, the HMO concept may also mean quicker referral to a specialist in a complex case. To illustrate, the primary care physician might incur expenses while struggling at the outer limits of his knowledge and experience, searching for the right diagnosis or an effective treatment, whereas an even higher-paid specialist could be more familiar with the presenting syndrome and get more quickly to the heart of the matter.

Alternatively, it may mean that the primary physician takes more *time* with each patient, thus lowering the most common yet simplistic measure of productivity, the volume of patients served.

Physicians work in HMOs for a variety of reasons, and not all physicians hired by HMOs have a realistic commitment to the HMO concept. They may "understand" it intellectually but not experientially. To fill in the gaps, the HMO can provide a formal orientation to its twin goals (good care, efficient delivery) so that the new physician develops a commitment to them that enables him to achieve both, thereby satisfying his patient's expectations and serving the needs of the organization as well.

Some formal orientation programs begin immediately and are extensive, thorough, and ongoing, with opportunities for continual, perhaps less formal reinforcement leading to a deepening of the commitment to prepaid medicine. Other orientations are rather minimal, little more than introducing a plan's forms and procedures without providing an opportunity to question or even challenge the plan's apparent values or develop a complete understanding of its operational meaning. It may be little more than what managers in more than one successful staff-model HMO reported to us, in almost the same words: "We hire the best docs we can find and turn them loose!" In some markets, that may be enough for a time, but it is not likely to ensure long-term survival of the organization, especially in an increasingly cost-conscious, competitive local environment.

### Arrangements for Hospitalization

Obviously, HMO physicians must have the capacity to hospitalize patients, even though studies show that the surest way for an HMO to contain costs is with low rates of hospitalization for its subscribers (Luft, 1987). The HMO may provide this capacity by owning its own hospitals, in which case it will keep the bed/population ratio relatively low, or it may contract with selected hospitals, promising an expected volume of admissions and patient-days in exchange for a favorable per diem price.

The care with which managers enter into these arrangements is important. The plan's good physicians need to have confidence in the quality of the hospitals. The prices need to be high enough that the hospital can live up to its end of the clinical bargain while the physicians know that financial allowances have been made for an adequate number of hospital days.

### Purchase of Supplies and Drugs

Similarly, the plan can offer a supplier a predictable volume of a drug in exchange for a favorable unit price. By doing this, managers give the physician a freer hand in exercising clinical judgment on most matters even though the choice of a particular drug is constrained. Failing to do so means the physician will feel pressure to compensate by further limiting other services. We note that at the same time the means by which the HMO's drug formulary is determined may affect the physician's attitudes toward management and the HMO and therefore his or her performance.

### Creation of an Efficient Record System

One of the elements of the HMO's efficiency is a clinical record system containing comprehensive medical data that are easily retrievable. With such a system in place, when the patient's regular physician is not available a covering physician will have the benefit of the patient's relevant history. Completeness requires that standards be established and enforced; retrievability may require automation, especially if services will sometimes be provided at a location different from the patient's normal site of care. Automated systems are expensive to introduce, however, and require continuous maintenance and revision. Even if they are a good investment, not all plans will be able to afford them. Purchasing or leasing a system (instead of building one from scratch) may make it more affordable, but there are obstacles to that solution as well. One is that it must be adapted to the HMO's current record system and to those of any new practices that join the plan. At any rate, this is another function that management undertakes with implications for how well the physicians are able to perform their role in providing good care efficiently.

### Creation of a Referral System

In a modern, integrated medical care system, many less common conditions can be treated most successfully and with expenditure of the fewest resources by highly trained subspecialists. The plan needs enough of them—either on staff or on contract—to serve their patients, but not so many that they sit idle or perform nonspecialty services that others could do with equal or greater competence at lower cost. At the same time, the plan needs a system by which primary care physicians can refer their patients to those subspecialists, and in which a consultation results in a useful service for the patient and feedback for the generalist.

One question to be faced is the degree of choice among specialists of a particular type; another is how the generalist selects the specialist in a particular instance. Choice is a good thing since competence is more than a technical attribute. The physician and the patient must get along in order for effective two-way communication to occur. Patients differ as to how much they want to know about their condition and the treatment options for it. Likewise, physicians differ as to how much information they are comfortable in sharing. Having enough referral capacity that in most cases a "fit" can be made is important.

It is also important that the primary care physician be able to choose effectively among competent subspecialists. In fee-for-service private practice, specialists and generalists have economic reasons to get to know each other: the specialist needs generalists who will make referrals to him, and the generalist needs to be able to refer to people he knows and in whose abilities he has confidence.

But in the staff-model HMO the same dynamics do not apply. A generalist may have little or no choice among urologists or gastroenterologists, for example. Where he does have a choice, he may not have had the same opportunities to get to know specialists as the ordinary fee-for-service physician does. He does not spend time with them in hospitals, partly because the primary care physician is not at the hospital much; and even when he is there, he does not have much time for building professional relationships in a system with limited capacity to subsidize nonclinical activities. (As an illustration, in a staff-model HMO, the generalist is not charging fees that in his own practice he might set high enough to permit him to spend a morning at a hospital's grand rounds.) If he has severely limited choices among specialists, or if he does not know them personally, the generalist cannot intervene as effectively in the event that a communication problem develops (as when the patient complains that he "could not get through" to the specialist or that he did not understand what the specialist was trying to say). Yet, being able to intervene in such an instance is one element of quality in an integrated system such as an HMO. It is up to managers to create conditions that facilitate effective referrals or that at least minimize the potential for dysfunctional relationships.

## Compensation of Physicians

The HMO is paid in advance and independently of the services actually used by patients. The HMO's ability to achieve its goals is affected by how the physician is paid and by the process by which managers determine the amount (that is, either unilateral decision or negotiation with individual physicians or with physicians as a group).

On a fee-for-service basis, even if some pay is withheld until year's end to protect against possible deficits, the financial incentives of the plan and the physician are at cross purposes. The physician earns more by providing more services, but the organization benefits when he provides less (though not "too little").

If he is paid a salary, the physician no longer benefits from providing unnecessary services. At the same time, although he still has professional and ethical standards to guide him, he does not have so great a financial incentive to work hard. Capitation payments made directly to physicians give them the same incentives as apply to the organization to do well in a competitive market, but an individual physician's practice may be too small to absorb the risk. The point is not that only one compensation method is appropriate; rather, the manager's task depends on whether or not the payment mode encourages physicians to provide services with only marginal benefits for patients.

In addition to the *method* of payment, the *amount* is an important consideration. The pay rate must balance the organization's and the physician's conflicting needs. The organization wants to keep its costs down, and physician compensation is an important component of those costs. The physician wants to earn an income that he can consider a suitable reward for his expertise and long years of training and that enables him to purchase those things he values (home, education for children, cultural opportunities). Missing that balance point can have serious implications for the physician and thus for the organization.

Finally, the means by which the compensation rate is set is also important and may affect the likelihood that the rate will fall in the correct range. Negotiation between representatives of the organization and the group of physicians is one method. Independent determination by the organization's managers of what they can afford to pay different groups of physicians and then imposition of their will on the physicians is another method. Negotiation with each physician individually, supposedly to reward or punish performance, is a third method. A physician may view any specific rate of pay differently depending on which of the three methods was used to determine it.

Again, the point is that care must be taken (Abel-Smith, 1988). This function too can be performed well or poorly by management, with important consequences for how successfully the organization achieves its goals.

This list constitutes a minimum set of critical managerial functions for a staff-model HMO; managers also perform additional activities. Each task may be performed well or poorly, but it is hard to imagine an HMO that is missing one or more of them.

It is also important to note that other types of MCOs whose gross income is predetermined like the staff-model's have some characteristics that require these functions to be performed differently from the staff-model. Nonetheless, most if not all of these functions will have counterparts in other forms of MCOs.

### Other Management Functions

Other functions performed by management in staff-model HMOs include:

- Creation and implementation of automated feedback systems using aggregated clinical data so that a physician can compare his patterns of clinical practice and their costs with those of his colleagues

- Routine annual (or more frequent) performance reviews that are formalized and include a standard set of measures and possibly some nonstandardized measures

- Creation of a corporate culture that reinforces the organization's values (responsive, effective, efficient care; informal consultation among colleagues; limited hospitalization; satisfied patients; and others)

- Creation and implementation of clinical algorithms or protocols to guide physician response to common presenting clinical problems

With all of these activities—the minimum set as well as the additional ones—management attempts to influence physicians' clinical behavior in order to achieve the organization's twin goals of providing care that is both effective and efficient. It is important to recognize that some, indeed most, of these methods are rather indirect. Only a few are or can be intrusive: for example, when the protocols become not helpful guides to practice but the standard practice; or when the physician is told what his response to the feedback should be instead of being able to come to his own conclusions as to how he should respond.

This discussion is meant to illustrate the kinds of tasks that health care managers must perform in all contemporary health care organizations operating under financial constraints. Important variations would be found in other models of HMOs or MCOs; in hospitals; in community health centers; in walk-in, store-front clinics; and in other health care organizations.

## Managers and Physicians: Summing Up

It appears that the contemporary health care scene in the United States is characterized by organizations in which managers have increasing reason to enter into the clinical province of medical professionals. Not only are they poorly prepared and in many cases reluctant to intervene, but their attempts to do so are often viewed as intrusions into the professional domain of a resistant group of physicians whose values and orientation are at odds with those of managers. Nonetheless, these two groups increasingly find themselves working as employees or contractors of the same organizations, with mutual interests coexisting with their differences. The challenge for both is to find ways to overcome the differences so they can emphasize what they hold in common in pursuing the goal of providing good, responsive care to patients without using excessive amounts of resources. We believe it is the manager's responsibility to lead the search for that common ground, but managers and doctors must arrive there together.

In the next chapter, we discuss our view of what a "healthy health care organization" should look like as a definition of the objectives the manager-physician partnership should attempt to achieve.

. . . . . . . . . . . . . . . . . . . . . . . . . . . . . . . . . . . .

# Moving Toward the Healthy Health Care Organization

## Identifying the Critical Challenges

### Coordinated and Compassionate Care

Jim Morris was spending a quiet Thursday evening in his living room with his wife Susan and college-aged son Steve when the chest pain began. Jim, who was having trouble catching his breath, asked Susan to call his physician. Dr. Johnson had been following Jim's care in a large staff-model HMO for more than fifteen years. Dr. Johnson was not on call but his colleague, Dr. Condon, knew from Susan's description that Jim should be seen right away. He advised them to go straight to the emergency room at Community Hospital.

Jim's pain subsided as Steve drove him to the ER. The emergency physician on call had already spoken to Dr. Condon, who had retrieved Jim's medical records from the HMO's information system. The ER physician did an electrocardiogram, which showed nonspecific changes, and ordered an immediate echocardiogram. By the time Jim returned to the emergency room, Dr. Condon had arrived and greeted him reassuringly.

"Well, you're having quite an eventful evening, aren't you? I know you're worried. Right now we don't have a definite diagnosis and your pain is gone, which is a good sign. But I think it would be best if you stayed the night for observation. We can see about next steps in the morning. Susan and Steve are welcome to stay, or we can call them at home if anything changes, whichever you prefer."

Jim spent a quiet but sleepless night on the telemetry unit and thought, as he observed the early morning bustle on the unit, that he must have imagined the chest pain the night before. Then it returned again, as painful and frightening as ever. He called for a nurse, who did an electrocardiogram while another nurse called Dr. Johnson. As it had the previous night, Jim's pain subsided gradually after about ten minutes. A few minutes later, Dr. Johnson entered the room and explained that, although there was no indication that either of Jim's chest pains had been a heart attack, he felt that further evaluation of a heart condition was warranted.

"The pain you had was not necessarily cardiac pain, Jim," the doctor said. "It could be due to indigestion or a gallstone or any number of other causes, but the most serious possibility is that you are having pain due to constriction of a heart vessel. We're fortunate to be a short ambulance drive from some of the best cardiac care centers in the country, and I think we ought to send you in to have a thorough evaluation. I'm going to call one of our cardiologists at Metro Hospital right now and the whole transfer should be taken care of within a couple of hours. Meanwhile, I'm right here."

Three hours after Jim was transferred to Metro Hospital, he was prepared for a cardiac catheterization procedure, which would assess the condition of his cardiac arteries. Before his procedure, the cardiologist, who had spoken at some length with Dr. Johnson and was now familiar with Jim's medical history, advised him that if a major vessel was found to be significantly blocked, it would be a good idea to perform an angioplasty, a procedure that involved threading a tiny balloon into the part of the vessel that was blocked and inflating it to collapse the blockage and open the vessel.

Jim consented to the procedure if it were found to be necessary. He awoke two hours later and was informed that indeed a major artery had been nearly totally occluded and an angioplasty had been successfully performed. Within a week he would be home and on his way to recovery.

The next morning, Dr. Johnson stopped by to visit Jim. "Nothing like a little excitement, is there, Jim? After a few days you'll be feeling a lot better. We'll keep a close eye on you for a while and I'll work with the cardiologist to make sure that your health care is coordinated properly between the general health issues you and I deal with and the cardiac care."

He stayed on a few more minutes to chat with Jim and to answer some of Susan's questions. Jim felt reassured that Dr. Johnson was there to "run interference" for him in this large and complicated medical center—and reassured that the resources of the health care system were called upon when they were needed.

◆　◆　◆　◆　◆　◆　◆

This vignette offers a picture of just how good health care can be in a complicated situation. There is evidence of a long-term and trusting relationship between Jim, the patient, and Dr. Johnson, his primary care physician. There is evidence that when Dr. Johnson is not available, Jim's records are readily accessible to Dr. Condon, who, although he is not Jim's primary care provider, is informed, communicative, and sensitive to Jim's understandable anxiety about his condition. There is evidence that first-level care is provided in a community setting by a capable primary care provider, but also that caution is used in a potentially serious situation. Further, there is evidence that Dr. Johnson recognizes the limitations in both his own clinical experience and the capacity of the community hospital in which he practices, and that he recognizes the advisability of transferring his patient to a more appropriate tertiary care setting.

Throughout Jim's saga, the physicians are caring, supportive, and informative. They advocate for Jim and for his family both in the community hospital where they practice and in the larger and more intimidating referral center. The care Dr. Johnson provides is both responsive and responsible. The care the system enables is informed, coordinated, and compassionate.

In this chapter, we begin the search for the "healthy" health care organization and attempt to define what characteristics such an organization ought to have. We try to draw a picture of an ideal health care organization from the patient's, the physician's, and the organization's perspectives, and to specify the challenges managers face in trying to create such an organization. We do not undertake this effort with the idea that there is only one way to achieve the goal of a strong and successful organization that delivers good services to patients. But there is evidence to suggest that several managerial and organizational capabilities are particularly critical to health care system success.

## Toward the Ideal Health Care Organization

We begin our quest for a healthy health care organization with the observation that *the primary goal of medicine is to provide for the health care needs of individuals*. The medical profession in the 1990s has the capacity, based on science and much recorded experience, to do a considerable amount of good for people: preventing illness, curing acute illness, restoring functioning in the aftermath of accidents, and managing increasingly prevalent chronic illness. But while its armamentarium has become more powerful, the processes of medical care have become much more complex. It is now quite common for even the most routine illness to require multiple tests, multiple treatments, and multiple drugs provided by a variety of people in several settings. As we have demonstrated, health care organizations increasingly constitute the site of care or the auspices under which it is offered. Therefore, the set of policies and systems by which those organizations operate is of critical importance.

Still, it is the physician who remains the key health care professional, and the growing complexity of medical care has given new meaning to the old expression that the physician's role is to be "captain of the team." It is likely true, however, that many physicians have not learned to act effectively in that role and do not especially enjoy it. We believe one reason is that physicians are often made responsible both for providing care and for maneuvering their patients through a complicated maze of interconnected health care system components, without benefit of policies and practices that facilitate the smooth integration of care.

## Physician-Patient Relationships

People value personal relationships with their physicians. One reason is that when people are sick, they are both vulnerable and anxious. They look to physicians, who know much more about most health-related issues, to help them understand their conditions. When physicians speak authoritatively about those matters, patients tend to rely on what they take to be expert opinions, especially if they know and trust their physicians. This normal tendency to depend on the physician's greater knowledge is magnified when physical and psychological illness is serious and patients are frightened.

Despite the fact that for many the health care setting has shifted from the private office of the neighborly solo practitioner to an organization, there is much evidence that patients continue to value their relationships with their physicians (Freidson, 1970; Mechanic, 1978; Rodwin, 1993). Moreover, it appears that physicians also value ongoing relationships with their patients, perhaps because they feel more in control of the situation when they know a patient's medical history and personal style, or perhaps because relationships with patients tend to reduce the complicated and risky world of modern medicine to a more human scale (Heineke & Davidson, 1993).

But strong, active relationships between patients and physicians do more than just make patients and physicians feel better. An important ingredient of effective medical care is patient compliance with treatment plans, which have become increasingly complex, yet the literature has for many years shown alarmingly large gaps in the extent to which patients follow physicians' instructions (Freidson, 1985). Among other things, patients report not knowing what they were expected to do. While compliance remains poorly understood, it is likely that a good and supportive physician-patient relationship helps patients comply with the physician's recommendations. It is also probably true that physicians, influenced by their relationships with patients, are more sensitive to reality factors that affect the ability of even conscientious patients to both understand and comply. If physicians recognize conditions that interfere with compliance, they may be able to adjust their instructions to take account of them. For example, when a physician encourages a mother of five young children to rest in bed, he or she may be able to define more specifically what "rest" means in that context and may even be able to suggest strategies for accomplishing it. A physician who has never seen the patient before and expects not to see her again, or a physician who feels like an anonymous cog in the medical care machine, is likely to be less sensitive to the patient's needs and therefore less able to help the patient work effectively toward her own best health. The physician may also be able to bring in other members of the medical care team. In the ideal health care system, strong physician-patient relationships built on a foundation of high technical quality would afford patients effective and efficient state-of-the-art care.

But even an ideal health care system would not exist without constraints. The costly secondary- and tertiary-level care that admittedly is needed in only a minority of instances would not be available in all locations. It would be the responsibility of primary care providers and organizations to maintain effective links with referral centers so that when the care required by a particular patient was not available locally, the patient could be connected with appropriate care at the next level *at just the right time: not too early, not too late*. Ideal health care would be *exactly* what the patient needs, when he needs it, in the most efficient site, administered by the clinically most appropriate personnel.

We use the word *ideal* recognizing that this may never be fully achieved. One reason is that medicine is as much art as science; in most clinical situations, no single action is the one best course to take. Rather, physicians may choose from several reasonable approaches to fit the condition and characteristics of the particular patient being treated. Even so, the ideal has heuristic value because it has identifiable attributes—timeliness, responsiveness, effectiveness, and efficiency—to which all health care professionals and organizations aspire.

In this context, we believe there are *two critically important roles for the managers of health care organizations:* first, to facilitate the establishment and full development of physician-patient relationships; and second, but no less important, to create policies and processes that promote seamless, coordinated patient care among providers, including nonphysician members of the patient-care team, both within individual organizations and across organizational boundaries. In such a system the care is personal, professional, efficient, and effective: sound, practical goals for healthy health care.

## The Challenges Facing Health Care Managers

To paraphrase the title of another book, a new management is needed to accommodate the "new medicine."[1] The primary challenge in today's health care system is to meet the health care needs of patients under contemporary conditions characterized by both complexity and constraint. An instrumental challenge for modern health care managers is to create, nurture, and maintain operating systems that produce smooth integration of the multiple services and of the people who care for patients in the organization—a task that should result in both lower costs and better outcomes of care. Part of the challenge is to foster the relationship between physicians and patients in a way that leads physicians to *act* for their patients, not just receive and respond to them when they arrive at an office. Physician action not only assuages the fears and concerns that patients feel when they or a family member are ill; it also promotes coordination and prevents the mistakes that can happen when communication is poor.

Patients and their families cannot be expected to manage their care during an episode of acute illness. They have neither the knowledge nor the objectivity to do so well, and as Heymann demonstrates through her many examples, they have trouble even making themselves heard (Heymann, 1995). Nor can physicians, even though they have the necessary clinical knowledge, be expected to negotiate the complexity of today's health care networks without systems, policies, and procedures to support them.

Managers focus primarily on the organization, a complex human system within a still more complex environment. Health care quality—in terms both of reasonable cost and best-possible clinical outcome—is the fundamental priority. To achieve an ever-improving level of quality, managers must develop systems for providing information on time and in forms that are useful to the physicians and other caregivers who make clinical decisions both within and across the organization's boundaries. Managers must also develop strategies for the use of medical and information technology to support effective and efficient care.

## Critical Capabilities

For a health care organization to be strong, the actions of its managers must engage physicians in defining the clinical challenges and opportunities that confront the organization, and in developing and implementing the policies and procedures that enable it to meet those challenges and take advantage of those opportunities. To do so requires the development of the capabilities of both the organization and its managers.

### Organizational Capabilities

An organization's capabilities are broad and are framed both by the mission of the organization and the way it chooses to compete in the health care market. Low cost, quality, flexibility, dependability, and service are competitive priorities that have been discussed in the management literature for some time (Wheelwright, 1984). It has long been believed that trade-offs between these priorities are inherent because, it is argued, organizations cannot succeed equally in all areas. In particular, it was believed that to achieve high-quality services required high expenditures and, of even more concern, that successful efforts to control costs would lead to diminished quality. However, better understanding of the relationship between cost and quality has produced both recognition that while good quality is not costless, poor quality has substantial costs as well (Berwick, 1988), and skepticism about any essential inability to compete successfully along more than one dimension at a time.

If we apply this idea of competitive priorities to health care, we can relate the ability to compete on the basis of *cost* to efficiency of care: whether resources are used and, if so, when and how they are used. There is no doubt that efficiency is important; the staggering increase in health care costs in recent decades has been central to health care's current crisis. The achievement of good *quality* is related to both process (conformance to standards of practice) and effective outcomes of care. Since we are unwilling to sacrifice quality to achieve low cost, any health care model must address each element in light of the other. To compete successfully on these dimensions in such a complex, changing environment requires organizational systems that are flexible yet dependable, systems that produce appropriate service.

*Flexibility* can be defined in several ways. First, it can mean the health care organization's ability to provide good care to a complex mix of patients: young and old, insured and indigent, worried well and seriously ill. It can also mean the ability to provide a wide range of services or to deal with many insurers. Most important, in the contemporary health care context, flexibility means internal systems that permit quick and timely adaptation to new regulatory and payer requirements and to diverse patient needs.

*Dependability* in health care implies access to care that is consistently timely, appropriate, and of good quality for all patients, not better for some groups than others or better at some times than at others.

One measure of *appropriate service* is customer satisfaction. The satisfaction of both external customers (patients) and internal customers (including physicians) should be greater when the system of care is efficient and the quality of care is high. When physicians are supported by the health care system, they will be better able to care for their patients. When patients have smooth access to care and seamless integration between specialties, they will be less frustrated and confused.

### Managerial Capabilities

An organization's ability to perform effectively along the critical dimensions of cost, quality, flexibility, dependability, and service depends on managers. None of these competing capacities can be achieved reliably without consistency between the goals of the organization and those of the clinical professionals who decide on the use of the organization's resources, especially those used in service of the primary external customer, the patient. As custodian of the organization, the manager has the responsibility to take the lead in developing that consistency.

Managers must also help physicians establish an identification with the organization as a whole and with its mission, instead of solely with the profession of medicine, or their specialty, or even their subgroup or unit within the organization. If we are right that for the organization to function most effectively physicians must identify with the organization as well as with their professional commitments, then it is the manager who must create the systems and processes that permit identification to occur and who must manage the tension inherent in the clinician's multiple loyalties (that is, to patient, profession, and organization).

## What Kinds of Organizations Can Meet These Challenges?

Any ideal model for categorizing organizational structures in the health care industry must consider the degree of physician involvement in management activities and the nature of the physician's relationship to the organization. Scott (1982) outlined three models of control for managing professional work in health organizations. His first two types, the autonomous and heteronomous organizations, are the "old" models for health care organizations. In the first, control over decision making (and therefore power) is held by physicians; in the second, by the administrators. In Scott's third model, the conjoint professional organization, clinical professionals and administrators have roughly equal influence. Neither group dominates; collaboration is the rule. The characteristic orientations of the physicians, who are concerned about the allocation of resources primarily in light of the needs of their individual patients, and of the administrators, who consider the acquisition and use of resources primarily in light of the organization's long-term health, are viewed not as obstacles to harmony but as legitimate perspectives needing to be voiced in decision making. Although airing these differing views produces tensions between the two groups, it also contributes to a fuller understanding of the complex health care issues, acknowledged by both groups to have both medical and managerial implications, and to their resolution in the service of patients and the organization's continued viability. The conjoint model can be visualized as a series of concentric circles, rather than as a strict power hierarchy.[2]

Scott's conjoint organizational model is intuitively appealing. It acknowledges the differences in the primary goals and orientations of physicians and managers in the health care system while making use of those differences to illuminate more clearly the fundamental problem: how to provide care that is both effective and efficient. By definition, collaboration is required for the success of a conjoint organization; joint policy decisions are based on the specialized expertise of both physicians and managers. Compromise results when both groups recognize that an acceptable, if not perfect, solution to most conflicts requires a set of legitimate trade-offs to reduce friction.

However, although Scott's model is appealing as an ideal form for organizations, it begs the question of how actually to resolve the real conflicts that can exist between the controllers of resources (the managers) and the users of resources (the physicians). The ways physician-manager conflict is manifested have been described by Bettner and Collins (1987) as dependent upon the physician's balance between the desire to satisfy his own concerns and his desire to satisfy the administrator's concerns.

Collaboration is the desirable orientation. Each decision made together reflects the specialized expertise of both physicians and managers. Both perspectives are recognized as legitimate, and so is the interactive face-to-face process for arriving at an accommodation.

But collaboration between physicians and managers has not been the norm, at least in part because physicians have functioned relatively independently of their organizations. Instead, physicians and managers have adopted mechanisms for managing the conflict between them. Avoidant or accommodative conflict styles result when physicians perceive conflict with administrators as no-win situations and choose either to ignore the situation or to give in. Competition results when physicians view relations with administrators as potential win-lose situations that they then seek to dominate, or when managers have similar perspectives.

This conflict-handling model has shortcomings, however, because it considers only how physicians relate to administrators. When the model is reformulated to incorporate the perspective of the manager so that both viewpoints are considered, the power relationships between the two groups are evident. Both physicians and managers can either dominate or avoid interactions with the other group, but these behaviors ignore the potential for better decision making that characterizes collaboration as the rule for interaction. Scott's autonomous model maps to the physician domination region; the heteronomous model maps to the administrator domination region. Scott's conjoint organization model falls in the collaboration region.

But collaboration does not happen by itself. Many obstacles must be overcome and many bridges must be built. Because of differences in training and in the focus of their disciplines, managers and physicians often have different meanings in mind even when they use the same words. *Malpractice risk* is a good example. Managers see the financial costs involved and think about how they can best be limited. Physicians, however, feel stress from the fear that they may harm their patients, the fear of reprisal, the fear of the loss of professional status, and insecurity in relationships with patients—all in addition to the potential financial costs for which they buy insurance. Unless each group understands how the other defines malpractice risk and accepts its concerns as legitimate, meaningful discussions are difficult. This is one small example of a communication issue, but it illustrates the magnitude of a commonly found gap and the need to find ways to bridge it effectively.

Trust is another key issue. Physicians and managers share a history of finger-pointing and blame. Physicians need to trust that managers will not prevent them from practicing medicine well. Perhaps even more, they need to believe that managers will help them to be more effective in making practice decisions by providing key information and creating systems that they as the central caregivers can depend on to serve their patients. Managers in turn need to trust that physicians will consider organizational goals to be legitimate and will treat managers not as nuisances or worse but as significant members of the caregiving team. For these things to happen, however, each group must *earn* the other's trust through the shared experience of working together to meet the organization's challenges. Unfortunately, judging from reported complaints from both groups, we believe that most health care organizations have a long way to go to build that trust.

## Managerial Tactics for Achieving Collaboration

Building organizational capabilities requires collaboration, and creating collaboration requires specific managerial actions designed to bridge the gap between physicians and managers. It also requires a willingness by both groups to put aside longstanding attitudes about the other and to be guided instead by the new experience of working together. We believe that managers must take the lead in this regard, and that a successful strategy for achieving this desired level of collaboration includes four basic categories of managerial tactics:

- Development of structures: the formation of physician–manager work groups or the employment of other mechanisms for involving physicians in decision making.

- Communication, which involves building a common language and a shared perspective on important issues, as well as creating opportunities for productive interaction and supporting styles of conflict management that are consistent with Scott's conjoint approach (Scott, 1982).

- Development of internal systems that facilitate the making of good clinical and managerial decisions, such as information systems, compensation systems, and quality review and assurance systems.

- Establishment through shared experience of an organizational culture based on trust, shared mission, and respected leadership. Such a culture is the basic framework for implementation of the other three categories.

Many health care systems employ the first tactic of forming policy-building and decision-making structures with representatives from both medicine and management. But even if physicians and managers are brought together to make joint decisions, they may in fact be unable to do so effectively because the other three elements of a successful strategy are missing. Building a common language and healthy communication is more difficult, primarily because communication must be established successfully before effective decision making can occur (since decisions are a product of purposeful communication); yet it is in the decision-making arena that constructive communication patterns either form or fail. The busy lives of both physicians and health care managers, as well as the financial constraints faced by the organization in a competitive environment, make it difficult to create opportunities to talk and understand each other even when the purpose is to make decisions on matters of importance to the organization. As a result the process may become circular, as old communication problems are reinforced by insufficient chances to resolve disagreements over issues that really count.

Similarly, the installation of information systems that are truly used to support good clinical care depends on productive communication in the design stage as well as with the fourth tactic, creation of a shared culture built on trust and an overarching commitment to a shared mission. Because the languages of medicine and management are so different, even a well-intended offer to provide clinically relevant information to caregivers is often met with skepticism born of the belief that managers are just trying one more way to impose constraints on professional practice.

While tested tactics for achieving collaboration do exist, it is critical to ask about the extent to which they are being employed and about where they are and whether they succeed in contemporary health care organizations. How well are health care organizations currently performing? These are empirical questions that can be answered with well-designed studies.

## Health Care in Organizations: Focus on Physicians and Managers

The health care industry can be examined at several levels. Most often, these examinations have been conducted either at the macroeconomic level (for example, how to finance the national health care system) or at the individual physician level (what it is like for a physician to practice the profession of medicine). We have argued here that the organizational level of analysis and the analysis of the interaction between physicians as a group and managers as a group requires more attention, but without losing sight of either the environment within which the organization functions or the relationships between physicians and patients that are its core.

Organizations have become the mainstream of the U.S. health care system, yet we know little about how they actually deliver care. It is no longer enough to count on the involved parties' working out their differences based on the relative power of each. Health care is too important for financial considerations to continue to dominate, as recent experience attests. We need to understand behavior in health care organizations more fully in order to develop effective strategies to achieve more reliably the two-part goal of delivering effective services efficiently. We turn to that task next.

# 6

## How Are We Doing?

### *Measuring Efficiency, Effectiveness, and Satisfaction*

We began the previous chapter with a story that demonstrated what sound, coordinated, empathetic health care looks like, which is how we want our own care and that of our families to be provided. That story was fiction. What follows are two true accounts of modern health care gone awry. One story has a happy outcome; the other does not. The first story should look familiar to yet strikingly different from the story that opened Chapter Five. It is in fact the true story from which the fictional "ideal" picture was derived.

• • • • • • •

### Unmanaged Care

Mrs. N., a 71-year-old widow, was at home with her daughter and grandsons on a Thursday afternoon when she began to experience nausea and chest pain. She was in basically good health, under the care of a physician she had been seeing for several years and with whom she was quite satisfied. She had no known cardiac condition, but her blood pressure was being controlled with medication. She and her daughter were both former nurses, however, and she recognized immediately that the nausea and chest pain might mean she was having a heart attack. The nearest hospital, a community facility where Mrs. N. used to work, was twenty minutes away. Her daughter drove her straight to the emergency room.

By the time they arrived, Mrs. N.'s pain had subsided, but as she entered the emergency room it began again. The emergency room physician took a quick but thorough medical history and ordered an electrocardiogram. It showed the kind of nonspecific changes seen with many types of pain. Still, the emergency physician was cautious and felt it would be wise to admit Mrs. N. for observation: "Dr. C. is an excellent cardiologist. I wouldn't recommend just anyone, but he is really terrific." Mrs. N. agreed and by that evening, she was comfortably settled on the telemetry unit. Later, after the cardiologist examined her mother, Mrs. N.'s daughter asked Dr. C. whether instead of keeping her at the community hospital it wouldn't be wise to transfer Mrs. N. to one of the large cardiology centers in the nearby city, but he said it was unnecessary at this point, since the diagnosis of cardiac disease had not yet been made.

Mrs. N. had a quiet night but experienced another episode of severe pain upon rising in the morning. Dr. C. ordered an echocardiogram, started intravenous cardiac drugs, and transferred Mrs. N. to the ICU. By this time, Mrs. N.'s son, Dr. N., a physician, had arrived on the scene. He questioned Dr. C. and agreed that for the time being the treatment plan was appropriate. Mrs. N.'s daughter spent that night in the hospital with her mother.

The next afternoon [a Saturday], after 29 hours without any discomfort at all, Mrs. N. began to have almost constant episodes of severe chest pain. Dr. C., who had seen her that morning, was covering for seven other physicians and had other patients in the ICU but was taking calls from home. Mrs. N.'s pain was increasing in intensity and duration, but there appeared to be no plan to do anything.

At this point, Dr. N. called his best friend, Dr. F., also a cardiologist, and asked for advice. Dr. F. agreed to speak with Dr. C. about the treatment plan up to that point. When he called Dr. N. back, Dr. F. made it quite clear that Mrs. N. was at high risk for a heart attack if she were kept in the community hospital setting with no intervention. He recommended a tertiary treatment center and a particular physician. Dr. N. called Dr. C. and requested an immediate transfer for his mother. Five hours later, during which time Mrs. N. experienced increasing pain — and her daughter found it increasingly difficult to get a nurse to respond to the call light — the transfer took place. It was 3:00 A.M. Sunday, more than twelve hours after the continuous pain began.

At the tertiary treatment center, Mrs. N. was evaluated by a cardiology intern and resident. By 7:00 A.M. she had been seen by a staff cardiologist, and a call was placed to the cardiac catheterization team to evaluate Mrs. N.'s condition. When the procedure was performed at noon, a 99 percent occlusion of a major vessel was found. An angioplasty was performed successfully. Mrs. N.'s recovery was uneventful.

◆ ◆ ◆ ◆ ◆ ◆ ◆

This story raises several health care delivery concerns. First and foremost, Mrs. N. was being held for evaluation in a hospital that could not provide the diagnostic services she clearly needed. As her pain intensified, Dr. C. was taking calls from home and made no attempt to go to the hospital to reevaluate her condition. When it became clear that Mrs. N.'s family was not satisfied with the technical quality of the medical care being provided and requested a transfer, even the nurses disengaged from her care. Whatever communication they were having with Dr. C., it was not enough to get him to return to the hospital even though the stakes for a woman of Mrs. N.'s age and history were quite high.

Why did Dr. C. keep Mrs. N. in the community hospital despite having been asked about the advisability of a transfer to a tertiary care center? Was he motivated by financial gain? Neither he nor the community hospital could bill for services after a transfer. Was he distracted by events at home? In some contexts, the care he provided might be justifiable—in isolated rural areas for example—but for a patient with worsening chest pain and with the appropriate technology less than a half-hour away, the decision to transfer appears to have been clearly warranted. What was the responsibility of the community hospital administration, which might have been held partially responsible had Mrs. N. indeed suffered a potentially avoidable heart attack and chosen to sue? Even without malpractice concerns, what were the ethical responsibilities of the medical and management teams? And what costs would have been incurred if Mrs. N. had suffered a heart attack at the community hospital? There is no doubt that her length of stay would have been longer, her care more complex, and her recovery slower. It is also not unlikely that her long-term recovery would have been less complete, that risks of further complications would have been higher, and that she would have been much slower to resume her normal activities—that is, if she had been lucky enough to survive.

Another true story raises similarly distressing concerns.

◆ ◆ ◆ ◆ ◆ ◆ ◆

### Uncoordinated Care

A middle-aged, middle-class man was taken by ambulance to the emergency room of a big-city teaching hospital after he called the physician covering for his primary care doctor. He was treated in the ER for a myocardial infarction and after being stabilized was admitted to a bed in the same hospital. He remained hospitalized for ten days and was transferred to an extended care facility (ECF) for rehabilitative therapy. On being examined by the physician in the ECF, he was told that following his discharge he should consult his regular physician for treatment of an ongoing irregularity. Dutifully, when he returned home two weeks later, he made an appointment with his internist for the following week, explaining the need for the visit to the woman who took his phone call. When he arrived for the appointment, his internist did not know the reason for the visit, so the patient explained again. The doctor examined him, did some tests, and asked him to call in a week for the results. When he called as requested, he was told over the phone that he should make an appointment with a cardiologist whose name he was given, because his internist thought surgery was indicated. Worried, the patient did exactly as instructed, and the specialist's scheduler was able to arrange an appointment for five days later. When he arrived for his appointment, however, the surgeon too did not know the reason for the visit. He conducted an examination, ordered some tests, and asked that he be sent the records from the patient's hospitalization and subsequent visits. A new appointment was scheduled for 14 days later. On the tenth day, the patient suffered a heart attack and died.

◆ ◆ ◆ ◆ ◆ ◆ ◆

This case, another true story, also raises a number of important issues. None of the patient's physicians knew anything of his prior experience. The primary care physician was uninvolved and apparently uninformed by the covering physician about his patient's cardiac problems until the patient arrived at his office for an appointment following discharge from the ECF. None of the physicians who thought the patient should have further care communicated with any other physicians. The entire burden was placed on the patient, who, although undoubtedly anxious and probably bewildered by what was being said to him, did exactly what each physician asked him to do. No one recognized his anxiety or addressed it. Clearly, the processes of his care were not seamless. In a classic example of medicine as a "consulting profession," each doctor acted as if his role were primarily, if not exclusively, to wait for a patient to appear in the office for a consultation and then to respond to the patient's questions and test results.

## Who Is Responsible for Patient Care?

In today's large and complicated health care systems, whose obligation is it—indeed, is it anyone's—to smooth the transitions among physicians and organizations involved in the patient's care? What should the role of the primary care physician be? What are the obligations of the physician who covered for him after hours? What should the responsibility of the attending physician in the hospital be? Or of the specialist? What steps need to be taken to assure beneficial results? How do they vary by setting? That is, how should the situation change if the patient is covered by an indemnity plan, a PPO or IPA form of HMO, or a network-model or staff-model HMO? Who has responsibility to make things happen right? Does anyone? Does that person change with the nature of the plan? Although we do not know for certain that the patient would have survived appreciably longer if his care had been different, we feel confident in asserting that no one who reads this story would want to be treated the way this patient was treated.

Given the new variety of financing and organizational arrangements that are coming to dominate the American health care system, a natural question is, what were the conditions under which this patient was given care?

We have posed the question to various groups who heard the story. Some say it must have occurred under the old fee-for-service system because the providers appear to be independent practitioners with no connection to one another, just like the physicians who treated the patient in the various settings in which he sought care. Others say that, on the contrary, ordinary fee-for-service private practice is the one setting that would *not* have produced these events. Precisely because the physicians *are* independent, this reasoning goes, they need to maintain good relations with one another. Specialists, like the cardiologist in the story, need primary care physicians, like the patient's regular doctor, to refer patients to them. Therefore, a good cardiologist would have communicated with the referring physician about the patient they shared, at least partly in the hope that the primary care physician would appreciate the respect a phone call or letter conveyed and would send other patients to him in the future.

This view is reinforced by those who point out that in an HMO the financial incentives inherent in prepayment produce an emphasis on providing fewer services and on expending fewer resources to deliver those services. According to this scenario, because they are costly, delays, extra visits, and tests would have been avoided.

But others argue that even though an HMO is prepaid and therefore has an incentive to use restraint in providing services, most IPA-style HMOs tend to exist on paper only. At this stage in their development, it is pointed out, IPAs tend not to have the systems in place to support those incentives but instead protect themselves against overspending primarily by withholding part of the physicians' fees. Most do not introduce management processes to ensure that independent physicians have the information about the patient that they need to provide good service; nor do the IPAs actively attempt to strengthen physician relationships with one another now that they no longer have the financial incentives to maintain the connections that the old fee-for-service doctors had. Therefore, these commentators say, the patient was obviously in an IPA-style HMO.

Still another group of observers adds that these events could not have occurred in a staff-model HMO because, although it is prepaid and therefore is governed by incentives that promote the reduced use of services, physicians in a staff- or large group-model HMO, or even in a network model, *do* have connections with one another (either as colleagues practicing in the same staff-model centers or as members of the group or groups that contract with the HMO). These connections exist even though their financial well-being is not so directly tied to their relationships with other physicians, as in fee-for-service. Moreover, in contrast to the *under*management of the IPA, these "more advanced" forms tend to have better information systems, institutionalized coverage arrangements, and contractual agreements with specialists that would avoid the difficulties described in the story.

Yet a final group were not quite sure because, although this last point is true—at least in the abstract—the reality is that the support systems tend to be in a relatively primitive stage of development in most cases. Further, as noted, since the physicians' compensation is independent of their individual practice, they do not build the informal relations thought to be important in ordinary fee-for-service private practice.

The disturbing truth is that these events could have occurred in *any* of the financing and delivery arrangements now found in the United States, from the ordinary fee-for-service indemnity-insurance model to the staff-model HMO. Good doctors, who might have intervened to change the course of this patient's care, can be found in any combination of arrangements. But no *system* is well-enough developed to inspire confidence that if one's doctor were not among the best, the *system* of care would include safeguards to compensate for his limitations or would produce the missing connections and smooth handoffs from one professional or organization to another. Indeed, in our view, *the primary challenge* facing health care managers over the next ten years is *to create and maintain exactly that system of care*.

## The Basic Structure of Systems of Health Care

In most health care organizations, at least two parallel structures have developed: the administrative structure and the clinical structure. In larger health care systems, the clinical structure may have multiple substructures: medicine, nursing, pharmacy, physical therapy, and social services, among others. Each of these structures tends to be organized as a classical hierarchy exhibiting unity of command and a defined span of control (Charns & Schaefer, 1983). What makes health care systems unlike other professional organizations in which professionals are "managed"—including academic institutions and law firms—is the linking of the parallel hierarchies at multiple levels and the need for frequent interaction and joint decision making in relation to both the direct care of patients and longer-term policy matters.

The primary purpose of health care organizations is to meet the medical care needs of the patients they attract. We have already noted that since managers are the custodians of these organizations, the CEO has ultimate responsibility for the organization's success in meeting this objective and the host of instrumental goals that make it possible to achieve the principal one. To meet that obligation, managers must acquire resources and introduce and maintain processes that support clinicians in delivering services effectively and efficiently. Since many patients require services from several people (including multiple physician specialists, lab technologists, X-ray technologists, physical therapists, and social workers), part of the managerial role is to develop structures and processes that promote the smooth integration of services from several sources. They must also oversee the creation of policies and procedures that result in judicious use of resources in the delivery of those services. Finally, they are responsible for the production and dissemination of information of many kinds (financial and clinical) that support clinicians in their delivery of services and that permit the managers themselves to monitor and control the organization's performance.

To achieve their goals of effectiveness and efficiency, health care administrators engage in activities to plan and control resource allocation and to monitor and control the operations of the organization. By *control* we mean that managers organize processes that systematically allocate resources and that guide the day-to-day delivery of health care services to achieve stated goals of responsive, effective, and efficient service. We do not mean to imply that managers perform these activities entirely apart from physicians, but only to emphasize that they are responsible for assuring the long-term viability and strength of the organization.

For their part, the role of clinicians is primarily to serve patients. Some physicians are also responsible for overseeing or coordinating the clinical work of other practitioners in order to maximize the responsiveness and effectiveness and to control the cost of services delivered to patients. The purpose of the formal professional structure within the organization is to monitor the credentials and activities of the professionals who work under its auspices, as employers or contractors, and to assure basic quality of care. Clinicians, usually physicians, may be responsible for quality management, for workforce scheduling, and even for some service production control systems, such as utilization review. Physicians have these responsibilities because the organization has delegated them, in recognition of the clinicians' technical expertise, in order to gain support for these activities from other clinicians, or because the clinicians have refused to relinquish them as their own professional prerogatives. As Charns and Schaefer wrote: "Too often in organizations—especially professional service organizations—the work of managers becomes disconnected from the basic purposes of the organization and does not include decision-making on delivery of services, which is left exclusively to the professionals. Often the focus of managers becomes control over resources, which is seen by the health care providers as conflicting with their [the providers'] work. Conversely, providers of services often feel that in such situations they have no responsibility for the use of resources" (1983, p. 13).

The dual hierarchy of most health care organizations evolved from the traditional roles of physicians and managers. While Scott's (1982) conjoint model of health care organizations offers an ideal vision of collaboration between those two groups, in the following pages we will examine the actual performance of real health care organizations.

## Examining Health System Performance

In Chapter One we showed that physicians are increasingly found functioning in organizations, and we argued that managers, as minders of those organizations, have good reason to influence physician practice. As custodians, they have ultimate responsibility for the organizations' viability, which depends to a considerable degree on how effectively and efficiently physicians and other clinicians deliver services. Physicians who are unresponsive to patients' needs and desires or are ineffective in meeting them may cause the organization to lose subscribers, and physicians who waste resources in the course of serving patients may jeopardize the organization's fiscal integrity.

It is tempting to believe, then, that when physicians practice within organizations they are better able to meet patients' needs because they are supported by an administrative structure, and that they are more likely to meet those needs at lower cost because the organization is being tended by managers who concern themselves with the efficient use of resources. Yet, there is abundant evidence—exemplified by the two cases presented at the outset of this chapter—that managers have been unable to reliably affect physician practice patterns to achieve effectiveness and efficiency. There is also ample evidence of a functional chasm between managers and physicians in many organizations: the two groups often have difficulty even speaking the same language and finding common ground for decision making.

At this point we begin to explore the performance records of health care organizations along several critical dimensions, notably (1) the satisfaction of managers, physicians, and patients, and (2) the quality of the care provided, including both the efficiency with which resources are used to meet the needs of patients and the effectiveness of organizations in meeting those needs. Our careful look at these measures indicates that all is not well within organizations. Managers continue to be frustrated with their roles in relation to physicians, even in the newer, more integrated organizational types. Physicians continue to feel indignant and confused about the pressures on their practice patterns from nonmedical stakeholders. Costs continue to rise steeply. The quality of medical care in terms of both health outcomes and customer satisfaction is often called into question.

We begin our exploration of organizational performance by looking at levels of satisfaction with health care from the perspectives of managers, physicians, and patients.

## The Manager's Satisfaction

Managers often feel stuck in their relationships with physicians. As Rohrer (1989, p. 7) put it, "All administrators know that they dare not appear to tell physicians how to practice medicine." But there are many levels of managers in modern health care organizations, and their perspectives are not identical. Heineke and Meile (1989) interviewed eighteen health care managers (nine senior-level non-physicians, five senior-level physician managers, and four non-physician department directors) to elicit their perceptions of managing in the health care industry. They found that managers' perspectives on the challenges they faced varied with their position in the organization. Senior managers felt limited by physicians who, they thought, did not see the "big picture." Midlevel managers felt caught between their administrative superiors and their clinical chiefs. Even though they recognized their roles as linking the medical and administrative hierarchies, they felt the strain of being pulled in two directions without having consistently effective mechanisms for bringing the two groups together.

Managers may actually contribute to their own frustration with physicians, however, in the way they tend to characterize physicians. Derzon (1988), for example, relates a story about hospital administrators seeking advice on how to deal with what he called "physician greed." Yet, although the administrators felt frustration with physicians who appeared to be concerned primarily with their own economic well-being, they had to admit that finances and economic issues dominated their own agendas, too, when dealing with physicians. By limiting their interactions with physicians to discussions of the economic dimensions of health care delivery, managers invite economically oriented responses. Yet by extending the sphere of their interest into clinical matters, managers risk being perceived by their physician colleagues as intruding into territory where they have neither expertise nor legitimacy.

The increasing responsibility managers have for controlling utilization and costs in the new health care environment amplifies the tensions between managers and physicians. To deal successfully with their new challenges requires managers to reduce those tensions, first by seeing physicians differently (as colleagues with different expertise and roles in the organization), and second by developing a set of techniques for engaging physicians and facilitating their performance in the service of patients and the organization.

## The Physician's Satisfaction

Managers are not the only players who feel stressed. Physicians also express concern and consternation about their roles in the evolving health care system. One physician wrote to *The New England Journal of Medicine:* "The psychic toll on physicians has been immense, and it has been inadequately addressed. The attempt to conscript and 'collectivize' the medical profession is at sharp variance with the individualism for which we were chosen by our medical schools and that was cultivated during our training. We now sense a confusion of goals. For whom do we work? Is it for the patient? For the health plan? For society? The investor? The smart shopper? And what about the poor?" (Alper, 1987, p. 339).

This physician expresses the difficulty many of his colleagues experience practicing in a system that has evolved to the point that organizational and financial considerations at times appear to preempt or dictate medical decisions. He also focuses the challenge faced by managers: how to create the practice conditions that maintain the strengths of "the old days," meet the efficiency and effectiveness goals of today, and create a practice environment that will be professionally satisfying for physicians tomorrow.

Physician satisfaction with practice in organizations must be viewed in the context of a dramatically changing medical practice environment, which is influencing decisions and attitudes of both the physicians and the organizations through which they deliver services. We imagine the process as a *series* of decisions, each of which develops from what has come before and influences what comes after. Although it is not possible to go back to the beginning of the chain—in a real sense no point has any meaning as a beginning—

the growing preoccupation with health care costs led employers in the 1970s to begin the search for new ways to provide coverage to their employees without committing themselves to the apparently inexorable, higher-than-inflation rate of growth in spending. Among other things, they changed insurers, choosing lower experience-rated premiums instead of renewing old policies; but as noted in Chapter Three, the reduced expenditures did not last long, and many began to turn to various forms of managed care: staff- and group-model HMOs, IPAs, and later, network models. Then PPOs were invented and began to flourish, leading some HMOs to respond by developing point-of-service plans in order to compete. Increasing numbers of the MCOs were organized for investors' profit.

At first, physicians could ignore these developments because relatively few patients were involved. But as the organizations grew, more and more physicians had to sign contracts with MCOs in order not to lose patients of long standing whose employers were giving them fewer choices. So, people were faced with a situation in which both patients and physicians were driven, by their employers' response to inexorably rising health care expenditures, into health care organizations in which most of them did not want to be. They were especially unhappy because although HMOs and other managed care arrangements can be justified on a variety of grounds, including the capacity to deliver better integrated and improved care, the clear impetus for the changes was the powerful search for reduced expenditures. The common fear was that patients would be denied services they really needed, and that physicians would be forced to practice cookbook medicine or, even worse, would be told by clerks at the other end of an 800 number what care to provide.

Generalized concerns over medical care costs, as well as specific controls imposed by insurers of all types, have both constrained practice and affected popular sentiments toward physicians as a group. "Most physicians believe that group practice is the best insurance against further attrition of professional prerogatives from payers and hospitals. . . . Increasingly, physicians will rely on physician groups or hospitals to help access a bewildered and fractured market" (Derzon, 1988, p. 12). While this comment reveals at least some degree of adaptation to new conditions, it is a reactive response energized primarily by an attempt to maintain old tactical positions in relation to organizations. The management challenge is to create new and more effective approaches: new systems of care that can satisfy the needs of both professionals and patients in the face of real constraints. It must be met even in organizations formed by the amalgamation of physician groups and hospitals (such as PHOs) and in those in which hospitals have bought established physician practices.

Measures of physician job satisfaction provide evidence that this challenge has not yet been mastered. Job satisfaction in industry is a well-studied field, going back at least to the development of industrial psychology in the 1950s and 1960s (Porter & Lawler, 1965). By the mid 1970s the field had come to recognize that job satisfaction is not a single concept but a complex construct (Porter & Steers, 1973). The scholars who produced this stream of social-psychological research had little interest in satisfaction among physicians until recently, primarily because so few worked in organizations, except perhaps temporarily during their training. As a group, physicians had autonomy, status, income, and other extrinsic rewards from their work, and it was simply assumed that satisfaction with their work was high. Only recently, as the changes in the environment that we have been discussing have become so prominent, did researchers turn their attention to physicians (Lichtenstein, 1984; Linn et al., 1986; Murray, 1988; Cashman, Parks, Ash, Hemenway, & Bicknell, 1990; Richardsen & Burke, 1991; Schulz, Girard, & Scheckler, 1992; Stevens, Diederiks, & Philipsen, 1992; Chuck, Nesbitt, Kwan, & Kam, 1993; Sutherland & Cooper, 1993).

These studies have begun to develop some strong measures of physicians' job satisfaction, which show repeatedly that autonomy and control are key factors in determining how satisfied physicians are with their jobs (Schulz, Girard, & Scheckler, 1992). Of particular interest is the work of Baker, Cantor, Miles, and Sandy (1994), which shows that among physicians in group- and staff-model HMOs autonomy was the most important factor in predicting practice and career satisfaction. Greater dissatisfaction was reported by physicians who saw themselves as having little control over their work hours, time with patients, and access to resources. Indeed, issues relating to the practice itself can be grouped as those embodied in the relationship between physicians and their patients and those growing out of the new relationship between physicians and the organization. Our primary interest here is with the latter.

Evidence of tensions in the relationships between physicians and managers attributable to these sets of issues is not new. A 1969 study by Ross found that physicians most often cited economic factors as the main reason for leaving large multispecialty group practices. Their managers, however, reported that physicians most often chose to leave for personal or family reasons. This discrepancy is an indication, going back more than twenty-five years, either of a lack of effective communication between physicians and managers or of managerial unwillingness to accept the physicians' actual reasons for leaving group practice. Physician dissatisfaction with their more limited income in group practice settings has been supported in other early studies as well. Prybil found that income was the leading cause of physician exodus from group practice settings in his 1971 study of 418 physicians. Second and third reasons were "too much supervision" and "lack of control over work hours," early evidence that physicians found managed settings constrictive. It is clearer now than it was then, however, that although MCOs continue to evolve, they can no longer be considered either a new or a temporary phenomenon. The stakes in physician relations with MCOs are therefore higher now than they were in the early 1970s. Physicians can no longer respond to their unhappiness with the arrangements by opting out of organizations altogether.

For some time, physicians have expressed dissatisfaction with other important aspects of their work lives in organizations. Excessive workload was cited by McElrath (1961) and Freidson (1973) as major causes of physician dissatisfaction in New York City prepaid groups. Freidson also found that many physicians expressed dissatisfaction with caring for patients who felt contractually entitled to and demanding about their care. The common denominator in these studies is that physicians were unhappy about conditions that, because they worked in organizations, were beyond their control. However, physician satisfaction with their own work lives may not be related to their feelings about their ability to practice good medicine in these settings. While some studies have indicated that physicians feel constrained by practicing in more controlled organizational settings, others have shown that they believe they can provide good care in a prepaid group practice even though other elements of life in the organization are not gratifying (Hetherington, Hopkins, & Roemer, 1975; Baker, Cantor, Miles & Sandy, 1994).

More recent studies show that many of these feelings and perceptions have persisted, even though the context has changed dramatically. Lewis and his colleagues surveyed members of the American College of Physicians about their satisfaction with practice in 1991. They found growing dissatisfaction with internal medicine practice among their 1,290 respondents, particularly related to concern over loss of clinical autonomy, increasing administrative burdens, loss of income, and threat of malpractice litigation. Like the earlier studies, they also found that more than 80 percent of respondents were satisfied with their relationships with patients and their professional challenges (Lewis, Prout, Chalmers, & Leake, 1991).

Reames and Dunstone (1989) tried to explore the reasons for physician dissatisfaction with practice by interviewing in depth nineteen randomly selected physicians in a Midwestern community who were not employed by organizations (except for a radiologist and a pathologist), but some of whom did contract to provide care for HMO patients. Seeking to discover how physicians define the problems they face in practice and how they attempt to solve them, Reames and Dunstone found that nine of the nineteen were unhappy, seven were happy, and three were ambivalent about their practices. One physician in the unhappy group felt that HMO practice pitted the physician against the patient, reducing the physician-patient bond to a business relationship and increasing the risk of litigation. An obstetrician felt that interacting with patients had become less satisfying than it had been in the earlier days of his practice, primarily because of the threat of malpractice. Those in the happier group expressed most satisfaction with their relationship with patients. Five of the seven in this group were primary care providers, and they focused on their own attitudes as the cause for their higher satisfaction levels. One of the physicians in the happy group stated that he knew the world around him would not revert to a prior state, so he had to adjust to the changes that were occurring. Another whose concerns had been focused primarily on the malpractice risk had developed a way to think about minimizing litigation risk as part of his patient encounter routine. Still another indicated that he kept medicine in perspective, considering it to be an interesting career but not all there was to life. This study again points to the importance of control as an issue. Physicians who recognized that "control" of one's practice in the old way of thinking—nearly total independence—was no longer possible developed new mechanisms for achieving acceptable levels of control in their own lives, with the result that they felt more satisfied than those who were unable to find such mechanisms.

One uncontrollable aspect of managed care practice is particularly disconcerting to many physicians: the patients' need to switch physicians when they switch insurance plans. Physicians are faced with frequent requests for transfer of medical records and often are not able to determine whether patients are dissatisfied with the physician's performance or simply unable to continue in the practice because of an insurance carrier change (Alper, 1987). This uncertainty adds to the stress physicians feel about physician-patient relationships.

Several researchers have looked for a relationship between organizational characteristics and physician satisfaction, thinking that some organizations by their very nature are less difficult for physicians to work in. Burns, Andersen, and Shortell (1990) found that physicians practicing in for-profit and nonprofit hospitals expressed greater satisfaction with clinical autonomy, with the hospital as a health resource for the community, and with their input to decision making than did physicians practicing in public hospitals. Private hospitals were found to exert fewer economic controls over physicians, and there was less conflict with physicians over autonomy. Larger hospitals also tended to exert fewer normative controls, and physician satisfaction was higher. Burns and his colleagues also found that older physicians were more satisfied and less likely to express conflict with the organization. But this study does little to explain what it is about the different organizational and physician characteristics that really affects physician satisfaction.

One plausible theory might be that physicians do not share the goals of the organization. Working within an organization requires some understanding of and commitment to both its goals and its day-to-day policies and procedures. The introduction to working within any organization is generally made through a formal orientation to the system. Yet, in a survey of physicians in a large staff-model HMO, Heineke and Davidson (1993) found that on average the physicians felt inadequately oriented to both HMO philosophy and procedure and to their specific roles within the organization. If their experience is repeated in other health care organizations, then one reason for physician dissatisfaction may be managers' failure to use the opportunity provided by a formal orientation to begin to socialize them to the organization's culture. Conversely, it is unlikely that an orientation will dissipate substantial disagreements physicians may have with an organization's goals, structure, or processes.

The day-to-day changes associated with practice in managed-care systems can also be frustrating for physicians. For example, many complain about the increased paperwork, which has been compared to that of Medicare and Medicaid (Rose, 1993). Physicians often consider the forms and precertifications to be particularly onerous because each managed care plan has its own specific documentation requirements, and as a result they must learn many sets of procedures.

*The Wall Street Journal* reported on a poll conducted by the American Medical Association that found differences in perceptions of medical practice between older physicians and their sons and daughters. When asked whether they would apply to medical school if they were in college today, physicians "age 35 and under said yes by nearly 3 to 1. In contrast, 45 percent of those 55 and older said they would not do it again" (Anders, 1990, p. A1). The group of parent physicians was particularly uncomfortable with insurers attempting to influence their practice decisions.

Physician dissatisfaction with medical practice is also evident in the trend toward increasing physician involvement in management, discussed in greater detail below. Many physicians claim that they are becoming involved with management activity because they are concerned that clinical issues, including quality, should be under the control of physicians. For their part, health care organizations recognize the potential value of having administrators who are also physicians and paying them somewhat more than they do physicians who only practice or other managers. Physician managers in HMOs are likely to have somewhat lower salaries than physician managers in hospitals but higher overall compensation due to bonuses (Wallace, 1987).

Although a number of studies address physician satisfaction in organizations, one key deficit is common to nearly all: there tends to be little or no discussion of the effect of the organization itself on the physician. As a result we cannot say how much of the satisfaction or dissatisfaction is related to practice within *any* organization and how much is related to *particular* structures or to the way a *particular* organization is managed. If health care organizations are both an increasingly prominent and permanent part of the landscape, then the issue for physicians and managers alike becomes, on the one hand, how to make practice more satisfying both personally and professionally, and on the other, how to increase managers' confidence in its contribution to the organization's viability.

## Patient Satisfaction

If still another important measure of health care performance is patient satisfaction, then it too must be considered in the study of physician–manager relationships in organizations. In addition to being a measure of performance in itself, the degree to which patients are satisfied with a health care organization will affect their future behavior—and the long-term financial strength of the organization.

Patient perception of care was in fact long omitted from discussions of medical care quality in any context because patients were generally felt to be unable to evaluate the technical quality of the medical care provided. Only 33 percent of physicians surveyed by National Research Corporation, a health care marketing research firm, believed that consumers could tell whether one hospital provides higher quality care than another, although 45 percent felt that consumers could judge the quality of physicians (Jensen & Larson, 1987). Instead of technical medical care quality, patients are believed to rely on factors that they *can* understand and assess, such as "bedside manner" and characteristics of the hospital food or the waiting times in the office. Patient perception, however, is now attracting increasing attention, both from managers, who are concerned with market share, and from physicians, who are concerned about the effect of dissatisfaction on both their incomes and their risk of malpractice claims.

Patients choose among health care organizations on the basis of a variety of factors, including cost and access. The managed care plans often offer somewhat lower premiums and what seems to be a bewildering array of service options, and employers may encourage employees to choose these less expensive plans by varying the employee's share of the premium cost. But "managed care plans often require both doctors and patients to change their approach to health care. As primary-care physicians try to do their part to hold down costs, patients may have to adjust their expectations about the range of care they receive" (Jacobson, 1993, p. 1A). When patients are dissatisfied with either the cost or the services provided by their health plans, or when their employers offer limited or different options in order to control costs, they may switch plans.

Switching insurers may necessitate switching physicians in order for service costs to be covered by the policy, yet relationships between physicians and patients are a critical part of patient satisfaction with health care organizations. Patients are more likely to feel anger and dissatisfaction with their care when they encounter new physicians in different systems than when they have a long-term relationship with a single physician. As a result, managers as custodians of the organization have an interest in the extent to which physicians establish strong, satisfying relationships with their patients. Thus, they should want to create conditions that facilitate the development of those relationships or at least do not undermine them.

Consideration of the satisfaction levels of the key players—managers, physicians, and patients—is clearly critical to evaluating the performance of health care organizations.

## Quality

Quality of care is another measure of performance that should be considered in any comparison of the practice of medicine in organizations and in the more traditional models where physicians are more independent.

Although no one disputes that quality of care is important, it can be quite difficult to define and measure. Lohr and her colleagues wrote: "Quality of care is a multidimensional concept reflecting a judgement that the services rendered to a patient were those most likely to produce the best outcomes that could reasonably be expected for the individual patient and that those services were given with due attention to the patient-physician relationship.

Implicit in the concept of quality of care is the idea that services should be provided in a cost-efficient and cost-effective manner, because unnecessary, excessive, or inappropriate services do not contribute to a patient's well-being, [and] may in fact be harmful and waste the patient's resources" (Lohr, Yordy, & Thier, 1988, p. 17).

If manager-physician relationships are working well, we can expect to see progress toward delivery of care that is both more efficient and more effective. But research has shown that progress along these dimensions has been slow.

## Efficiency

Efficiency in health care can be defined as the degree to which optimal results are achieved with the least expenditure of health care resources. Studies have reported mixed findings on the cost of providing health care in organized settings. Hurdle and Pope (1989a) used data from surveys conducted by the National Opinion Research Center and the Health Care Financing Administration to study physician productivity. They found a substantial decrease in physician productivity over the decade 1975–1984, primarily in office visits per hour rather than in hours worked per year. Their study did not demonstrate higher productivity of HMO physicians than of those in private practice. Recognizing that physicians in private practice also care for IPA and PPO patients, they controlled for the proportion of each physician's practice that those patients represented and still found no difference. Hurdle and Pope also noted that physicians on salary or in large group practices tended to work fewer hours per week and per year than physicians in solo practice or in small group fee-for-service practice. Physicians in private practice, then, saw more patients in a year than physicians in large group practices, which might be related to the fact that physicians in fee-for-service practice expect to earn higher incomes when they see more patients, whereas physicians in group settings may not.

Although the fee-for-service physicians may be earning higher incomes, these results do not mean that private practice physicians are more productive than physicians in large group practices. But if they see more patients than salaried physicians in large group practices, it does signal to managers that their employed physicians may be able to see more patients in a given work day than they have been seeing. (In Chapter One, we cited reports that although physicians in organizations see fewer patients than those who work in their own small offices, they may be working long hours nonetheless, in part because of increased paperwork or activities associated with their role as managers of a patient's care.) If at the same time managers can keep the physicians' income fixed, then the organization will have produced more services for the same physician cost—in economic terms, that is higher productivity. If physicians are working substantially harder without benefiting directly—so that the organization can increase its margins—it is not hard to imagine that their satisfaction with their work would decline and that their relations with the organization and the managers who exacted this price would sour.

Conversely, managers do have a legitimate interest in physician productivity. The cost of care is an important consideration in setting the prices the MCO can charge subscribers and is therefore a factor with which consumers can differentiate MCOs. The question is thus not *whether* MCO managers pay attention to productivity but *how* they deal with physicians about it. Moreover, not only their sensibilities are at stake for physicians but also two of the most important professional goals: practice autonomy and income.

To study mechanisms employed to integrate physicians in hospitals, Alexander and Morrisey (1988) used data from the 1982 American Hospital Association (AHA) Survey of Hospital Medical Staffs, the 1982 AHA Annual Survey of Hospitals, and the 1982 Medicare Case Mix Index. They looked particularly at the employment of physicians in general administrative roles, physician participation in hospital governance, the employment of physicians to provide care in both hospital-based and nonhospital practices, and medical staff committees established for planning or cost containment. Controlling for other cost function variables such as case mix, Alexander and Morrisey found that hospital costs rose with an increasing proportion of physicians on salary and with increased involvement of physicians in general administrative roles. They caution that these integrative strategies may have benefits in terms of quality, revenue enhancement, or hospital/medical staff relations that must be weighed against the increased costs, and that conclusions should be based on the relative costs and benefits of physician integration.

Luft (1985) stated the crux of the issue succinctly. Although HMOs are more efficient than other delivery systems, price, not cost, will determine the benefit of this efficiency to enrollees. HMOs have had little incentive to offer their services for dramatically lower prices than their indemnity-insurance competitors even if their costs were low enough to support such a pricing strategy. As a result, they have been under less pressure to reduce their costs and there has been some question regarding the extent to which the cost savings they do achieve benefit society or the HMOs themselves. When market pressures force HMOs to concentrate more seriously on price (and thus on cost), the relationship between physicians and managers will be put to a tougher test. The nature of the organization's response to those financial constraints will determine whether physicians and patients alike are content with the new health care system.

### Effectiveness

Effectiveness can be defined in many ways. Most broadly, health care is effective when the patients' health-related needs are met. Though this is an appealing definition, its generality makes it difficult to examine directly.

Effectiveness of medical care is often framed in terms of clinical outcomes, but the relationship between the service and the postcare result is notoriously hard to measure because of the many patient-related and treatment-related factors that must be considered. Flood and her colleagues (Flood, Scott, Ewy, & Forrest, 1982) studied the relationship between organization and quality in fifteen acute care hospitals nationwide. They concluded that higher proportions of contract physicians and greater degrees of surgical specialization were associated with higher quality; but higher cost, measured as expense per patient-day, was also associated with higher quality. This finding is consistent with the work by Alexander and Morrisey cited earlier and begins to answer their question about what benefits are reaped as costs rise when physicians are employed. But again, market forces were very different when those studies were conducted, and how the various players would act under greater constraint remains an open, as well as critical, question. Could the same level of quality be produced with lower costs if market conditions demanded it? If so, how can managers best attempt to influence physicians to achieve that result?

Some studies have attempted to use specific clinical outcomes of care as quality measures, but it is difficult to control for the many variables that affect outcome in order to permit comparability across systems. Obstetrics is an attractive diagnostic entity for such studies because there is little disagreement as to the beginning and end points of pregnancy, and there is a high degree of comparability because the outcomes are either vaginal or cesarean births. Goyert and his colleagues (Goyert, Bottoms, Treadwell, & Nehra, 1989) examined cesarean section rates and found a very high degree of variation among physicians (from 19.1 percent to 42.3 percent), which probably indicates both a quality problem (that is, risk introduced by the variation in the way care is provided) and opportunities for improvement. (According to the same authors, tonsillectomy rates investigated in the 1960s showed dramatic variation by physician, and feedback and other forms of education were important in changing physician behavior and reducing the highest rates.) Heineke (1992), in a study of obstetric outcomes and management decisions in HMOs, also found great variation in cesarean rates.

Some systems were clearly more effective at controlling cesarean rates and thereby reduced the average costs associated with the delivery of a healthy baby. The effectiveness seemed to be related to whether managers attempted to manage the caregiving process at all or simply left the professional physicians to practice as they saw fit.

We have shown that there is considerable room for improving satisfaction with the current system for managers, physicians, and patients; that health care systems are not as efficient as they could be (and may need to be in the future); and that effectiveness of care, while admittedly difficult to measure, also appears to fall short of ideal. Managers are certainly aware of these results and have employed various tactics to improve organizational performance. We turn now to an overview of those tactics and an assessment of their success in achieving improvements in performance.

## Managerial Strategies for Enhancing Performance

Organized health care systems have attempted to improve both customer satisfaction and quality by reducing variability of practice through a variety of mechanisms, including clinical guidelines, financial incentives, feedback and education, and the employment of physicians as managers. The following pages outline the effects of some of these strategies for influencing or controlling physician behavior. (For a more extensive review that is now ten years old, see Eisenberg, 1986.)

### Clinical Guidelines

Lomas et al. (1989) reported in the *New England Journal of Medicine* that although physicians' *perceptions* of their practice patterns altered significantly two years after exposure to clinical guidelines, actual practice patterns changed very little. Physician and organizational attitudes were positive, however, and physicians appeared to have changed their views of what acceptable practice entailed. The researchers found that clinical guidelines more readily affected physician awareness and attitude than actual practice patterns.

Some organizations attempt to reduce practice variability by developing and using specific practice protocols. A fairly new variety of protocol is the clinical algorithm, which identifies key decision points and the choices for physicians to make along the path of a work-up for a particular problem or medical entity. For example, an algorithm may define how to manage the results of a routine annual Pap smear. If the smear is negative (normal), the patient might be instructed to return for another routine smear in a year. If the smear shows inflammatory changes, the next step in the algorithm might be to treat the cause of the inflammation and then repeat the smear in three months. If more serious abnormalities are found on the routine smear, the next step in the algorithm might be to perform a colposcopy and a directed biopsy of suspicious areas.

Heineke and Davidson (1993) found that although physicians in a staff-model HMO liked participating in the development of clinical algorithms, they did not particularly like using them, nor did they feel that algorithms were particularly important for improving clinical care. Conversely, the opportunity to think off-line about the steps in providing care and to review the recent literature seemed important to physicians, and perhaps to outcomes as well. For example, physicians at Duke University Health Services developed guidelines for all providers to use in assessing and treating acute pharyngitis, though they expressed the belief that protocols were most appropriate for use by nurse practitioners and physician assistants. Practice patterns of all clinical providers were assessed before and after the development of the guidelines, and *physician* practice was found to change dramatically along all of four key dimensions, conforming to the protocols and providing both more appropriate and more cost-effective care (Grimm, Shimoni, Harlan, & Estes, 1975).

The use of guidelines, it seems, can be an effective tactic for improving the delivery of medical care. But what may be more important is that algorithm development offers an opportunity for physicians to study the literature and to think, away from the demands of practice, about how to provide care.

## Incentives

Organized health care delivery systems have also used financial incentives to attempt to affect clinical efficiency and effectiveness. The basis for employing financial incentives has been the underlying belief that physician practice decisions are influenced in part by monetary considerations (Davidson, 1982).

In fee-for-service medicine, other things being equal, physicians have financial incentives to provide both a greater volume of services and more complicated services because both produce higher incomes for them. The relationship of physicians to an HMO is more complicated. When physicians are employees, they usually do not face specific individual financial incentives to perform services of either greater or lesser complexity or cost. In staff-model HMOs, for example, individual physicians are unlikely to have their salaries or bonuses tied directly to their own individual practice patterns, although it is not uncommon to have salaries and bonuses related to group or specialty performance. To date, fee-for-service is still the predominant method of payment for specialists in IPA systems (Berenson, 1991) and for all physicians in PPOs, although as organizations the IPAs and PPOs also seek to conserve resources and control costs. The incentives for physicians and the goals of the organization may therefore, in these instances, directly conflict. In such circumstances, other measures, such as using physicians as primary care gatekeepers and requiring prior approval for tests and procedures, are often instituted to control resource utilization. While these measures have indeed controlled some costs, they have often frustrated physicians, who feel they no longer have the freedom to practice as they see fit and who may resent nonclinical people passing judgment on the appropriateness of their medical decisions. Patients as well have felt alienated because the direct relationship with the physician has been either replaced by the relationship with the insuring organization or structured in a way that makes the step requiring primary care approval feel more like an administrative burden than a clinical consultation.

The role of financial incentives in affecting behavior has been studied extensively. Hillman published a special report in *The New England Journal of Medicine* on their use for physicians in HMOs and concluded that "certain financial incentives, especially when used in combination, suggest conflicts of interest that may influence physicians' behavior and adversely affect the quality of care" (1987, p. 1743). Hillman found that the incentive structures tended to differ by HMO type[1] and that older plans were more likely than new plans to use penalties in combination with positive incentives. He hypothesized that either the older plans had more leverage over physicians or the newer plans were more sensitive to the possibilities of inappropriate alteration of physician practice patterns through strong financial incentives. A third possibility is that newer plans needed to solidify their relationships with physicians because enrolling large numbers of new subscribers was a priority, and a large list of physicians is an important recruitment tool. Regardless, Hillman expressed concern about the use of strong financial incentives when the number of physicians in the group was small and the effect on an individual was likely to be substantial, but the ability to measure changes in practice was limited and technically difficult.

In a subsequent study, Hillman, Pauly, Kerman, and Martinek (1991) surveyed HMO managers about their perception of the effect of withhold accounts and bonuses on practice. Two hundred sixty-five HMO managers (44 percent) responded. Results indicated their belief that "the impact of withhold accounts, bonus payments, and risk pools are subject to thresholds below which little or no effect is expected" (p. 217) and that "quality assurance mechanisms would be likely to reduce the adverse impact on quality that with-hold accounts or bonuses could have" (p. 214).

When Medicare introduced the prospective payment system (PPS) and diagnosis-related groups (DRGs) in 1983, hospitals were motivated to reduce costs and lengths of stay (but not admissions). Since the incentives affecting the clinical decisions of physicians practicing fee-for-service medicine were unchanged, hospital man-agers needed to use other methods for bringing physician caregiv-ing decisions in line with the hospital's new interests. Most of their efforts in that regard focused on reducing length of stay.

Hemenway, Killen, Cashman, Parks, and Bicknell (1990) showed that physicians in a for-profit clinic increased the rates of ordering lab tests by 23 percent and radiographic tests by 16 per-cent during a three-month period compared with the same three-month period a year earlier after a program was established providing financial incentives to do so. Despite the increases, upon review of medical records the authors stated that they found little evidence of overtreatment.[2] This finding indicates either that the range of acceptable practice is very wide or that, as a method, med-ical record review does not readily permit identification of "over-treatment." In any event, incentives may differ considerably among physicians practicing within organizations such as HMOs, and their effects may vary. Further, we already saw that formal physician ori-entation to the goals and practices of those organizations may be insufficient to produce a change in the physician's point of view or practice behavior.

Feedback and training are other strategies that may be employed to attempt to increase the congruence between the goals of the indi-vidual practitioner and the organization.

## Feedback

By providing a physician with information comparing his own prac-tice pattern to those of other physicians in the same specialty in the same HMO, feedback may, for example, reduce variability in the organization by encouraging physicians to change their decisions. The use of feedback as a means to influence practice has been advocated in the literature for some time (Restuccia, 1982; Restuccia & Holloway, 1982) and has been shown to be effective (Payne, Ash, & Restuccia, 1991). Berwick and Coltin (1986), among others, reported that when feedback of test-ordering behavior was provided in a staff-model HMO, a decrease of 14.2 percent in overall test ordering resulted. But Heineke (1992) found in her survey of HMOs that although clinically useful data were often collected, managers reported that feedback was not consistently provided to physicians. In her study of cesarean section rates in HMOs in 1988–1990, 80 percent of staff-model HMO managers, 77 percent of group-model HMO managers, 48 percent of network-model managers, and 65 percent of IPA managers responded that feedback of cesarean information was provided to physicians. On average, feedback was provided only four times per year, and only half of the respondent managers believed that the feedback influenced physician behavior moderately or highly. Regardless of perceptions, however, feedback of cesarean information was not associated with lower cesarean rates. These results raise a number of questions, including whether some methods of providing feedback work better than others. Since there is evidence to indicate that feedback *can* affect clinical behavior, to what extent have health care organization leaders actually used it? What factors determine manager actions in this regard? While feedback has been shown to have some promise for affecting clinical practice, to date the long-term effect on practice behavior has been disappointing.

## Education

Another mechanism for improving customer satisfaction and quality in health care has been the use of continuing medical education programs. Continuing education is predicated on the belief that when physicians know what constitutes good care and how to provide it, as professionals they will do so.

Martin, Wolf, Thibodeau, Dzau, and Braunwald (1980) studied the effect of different interventions on test-ordering behavior by randomly assigning medical residents to three groups. The first group was offered a small financial incentive (to be used for educational purposes) to reduce test ordering. The second group met weekly with investigators to review charts, and the third was a control group exposed to no intervention. Both intervention groups reduced test ordering, but the reduction was greater in the chart-review group. Moreover, only the chart-review group sustained the reduction after the experiment ended. While endorsing education as a means to change behavior, Goldman wrote, "Unfortunately, competing forces—society's interests, patients' real or perceived demands, financial incentives, and fears of embarrassment or accusation of malpractice, to name just a few—also have a powerful influence on behavior" (Goldman, 1990, p. 1524). Citing several studies that demonstrated positive physician practice pattern changes, Goldman also advocated the use of other methods: administrative strategies, incentives, penalties, and feedback about current performance. Further, he stated that the absence of agreement regarding the benefit of testing makes it difficult to measure and interpret test-ordering behavior.

Continuing medical education, then, offers some potential for improving clinical care, but studies have shown mixed results and benefits that fade with time. This tactic is more likely to be acceptable to physicians, however, as it supports their autonomy as professionals.

## Clinicians as Managers

Physicians have become involved in the management aspects of health care organizations for many reasons, among them to gain greater control of decision making, to protect the profession from lay domination, to reduce costs because of greater understanding of management's goals, and to promote understanding of the problems facing the organization as a whole (Schulz, Grimes, & Chester,

1976). By 1993, the American Academy of Medical Directors was growing by 100 members per month, and the American College of Physician Executives had a membership of 7,300, up from 4,300 only five years before (Sherer, 1993). Physician CEOs typically earn 10 to 25 percent more than their nonphysician counterparts in similar organizations. Kindig and Lastiri-Quiros see the role of the physician manager as spanning the boundary between physicians and nonclinical managers. They argue that general management skills should be supplemented with clinical management skills that would include academic treatment of "quality assurance and measurement, cost-benefit and clinical decision analysis, technology assessment, management of professionals, community health needs from an epidemiological perspective, clinical and managerial ethics, and external and political relationships" (1989, p. 45).

Fox, Heinen, and Steele (1986) discovered that all eight of the "successful" HMOs they studied employed physician leaders in boundary-spanning roles between other physicians and managers. In addition, all of the plans recognized the importance of continued practice for these physician leaders as a way to maintain credibility with their physician peers. The degree of managerial responsibility of the physician leaders varied considerably between organizations, however. Some HMOs gave physician managers full responsibility for management of operating units, whereas in other HMOs physicians were limited to the more traditional clinical leadership positions.

Although supported by little empirical evidence of the effectiveness of physician managers in the roles outlined here, proponents and opponents of physicians as managers have argued their positions with intense conviction. The limited research to date has generated conflicting findings. Some authors have found that promotion of clinician managers can lead to reduced efficiency and effectiveness, increased costs, and morale problems, while others have found that clinicians with management training are able to improve organizational performance along these same dimensions.

As noted earlier, Heineke and Davidson (1993) found that physicians in a staff-model HMO tended to view physician managers more as managers than as physician colleagues and felt some distance from them. Part of the reason may be physician manager discomfort in the role of manager, which in turn stems partly from their lack of education and experience as managers. Tabenkin, Zyzanski, and Alemagno (1989) offered support for that view, concluding that training was the key variable in determining the degree to which physicians felt competent as managers: physician managers were both more involved in the organization and more satisfied with their managerial roles when they had more management training.

Betson and Pedroja (1989) found that the tasks for which physician managers tend to be responsible are consistent with what the literature suggests would maximize their influence on the efficiency and effectiveness of their organizations, particularly their involvement in policy development. Specifically, they identified coordinating, conflict management, and organization decision-making tasks as in the realm of physician managers, but they identified financial management as usually outside physician control.

Involving physicians as managers as a tactic to improve organizational performance, like the tactics discussed in the preceding pages, has shown mixed results. While it supports the role of the physician and provides a more effective means to span the boundaries between physicians and managers, there is little empirical evidence that organizational performance does indeed improve, or even that clinicians are more satisfied with their work in organizations that employ physician managers.

## Summary

In this chapter we have demonstrated that the increasing trend toward delivery of health care services in organizations has exacerbated long-standing tensions and strains between managers and physicians and has not reliably improved efficiency or effectiveness or the satisfaction of either patients or physicians. In fact, some studies show results that are opposite to those desired. We have also reviewed some of the tactics that managers have employed to improve efficiency, effectiveness, and satisfaction and have found them lacking, primarily, we believe, because they *are* tactical rather than integrated elements of a comprehensive strategy. Their mixed results have led to more questions about how best to manage systems as complex as health care organizations.

Yet the need for answers to those questions becomes more urgent with each passing day. What does it take to develop a system for practice in organizations that will enhance both performance and satisfaction? What should the organization expect of the physician—and what should the physician expect from the organization—to make performance stronger? In the next chapter, we offer a framework for research to answer these questions.

# Understanding the
# Physician-Manager Relationship
### *Five Perspectives*

Having demonstrated the importance of organizations in the delivery of health services, we argued that productive collaboration between managers and doctors is needed for those organizations to succeed in their core activity of providing health care services. We then showed that physicians and managers have had a history marked more by antagonism or avoidance than by collaboration. Before we can identify an approach that can be used to develop a more productive partnership, we need to understand why their relationships have been so difficult in the past. We turn to that task in this chapter.

Here we summarize the attempts of researchers and other observers of the health care system to explain the difficult relationships between physicians and managers in health care organizations. The goal is not just to review relevant academic perspectives but more importantly to summarize a variety of viewpoints on the *causes* of the traditional difficulties in physician-manager relationships in order to provide a framework that can help practitioners find ways to improve those relationships.

Our review produced two broad findings of interest: first, most researchers have not tackled the subject of physician-manager relationships empirically. In fact, many writers discuss the health care system *assuming* that physicians and managers will always work in conflict with each other, without demonstrating why that should be the case. Second, we found that while some researchers have looked extensively at the ways that relationships between groups of physicians and health care organizations are structured, there has been little empirical research and analysis of the relations between physicians and managers *within* specific health care settings.

These observations reaffirm our conviction that, as important as physician-manager relations have become, scholars have not provided a solid empirical foundation either for understanding current relations between physicians and managers or for developing effective strategies to improve them. To make progress toward these ends, we must:

- Understand the causes of problems in the physician-manager relationship

- Develop a model of health care organizations to show the circumstances under which cooperative relations between physicians and managers are possible in those settings

- Understand how effective health care managers—from the supervisory level to the CEO—can bring this model to life

We undertake these three tasks in the last three chapters.

We have organized the review in this chapter by identifying five quite different perspectives on the topic and by discussing the view of physician-manager relations offered by each body of thought.

The *contextual* perspective considers government policy and competition in the market to be the primary drivers of change in the health care system. The ability of physicians and managers to cooperate is seen to have been compromised by recent changes in those dimensions, which occur in the environment external to the organizations.

The *professional* perspective views physicians and managers as members of large social classes or professions. From this perspective, individuals' behavior is influenced primarily by their socialization and membership in these powerful professional peer groups rather than by their roles in specific health care organizations.

The *organizational* perspective focuses on the unique characteristics of health care organizations, which implicitly render them extremely difficult to manage. Problems in physician-manager relationships are created by the complexity of the organizations' tasks and by limitations in managerial competence.

The *intergroup* perspective sees physician-manager tension as the product of the conflict that inevitably occurs between interacting groups *within* an organization. Unproductive behaviors are caused by conflicts over the way work is structured in particular work units, departments, or subspecialties as well as by the different priorities and perspectives of each group in the organization.

Finally, the *individual* perspective proposes that self-selection into careers by personality type is the root of difficult relations between the two groups. From this perspective, physicians and managers would in general be expected to reveal widely varying profiles on personality inventories.

The relationships among these five perspectives are illustrated in Figure 7.1. In the rest of this chapter, we discuss each of them in turn, considering (1) the argument *for* that particular explanation of the difficulties in physician-manager relationships, (2) how extensively this view is represented in the literature, and (3) managerial strategies that might be, or have been, employed if this explanation were correct. We also explore the differences among the five perspectives.

## The Contextual Perspective

The dominant perspective in the health administration literature of the last twenty years is the view we call contextual. The theory behind this perspective is that the unsatisfactory relationships between

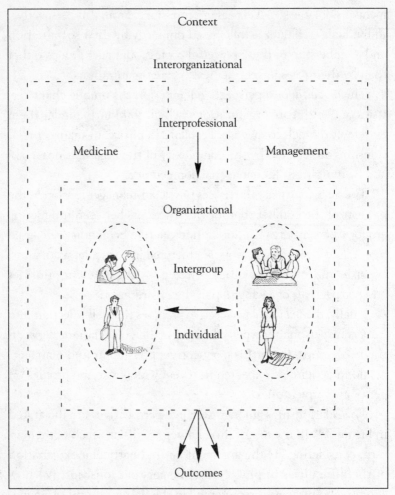

Figure 7.1. Levels of Analysis for Understanding
Physician-Manager Relationships.

physicians and managers in health care organizations, evidenced by
the suboptimal performance described in Chapter Six, result primarily from a series of dramatic changes in the environment in
which medicine is practiced, that is, from changes in the economic,
institutional, societal, and political contexts of the professions.

Some researchers in this group have focused on the introduction of Medicare's prospective payment system (PPS) in 1983 as the
single most important event reshaping (and damaging) the rela-

tionships between physicians and managers in hospitals (Burns, Andersen, & Shortell, 1990; Glandon & Morrisey, 1986). For example, Burns and colleagues summarize the impact of the prospective payment system as follows: "[P]hysician-hospital interdependence has become more competitive. . . . Competitive interdependence between physicians and hospitals thus generates tensions that may not be restrained by traditional conflict resolution strategies" (p. 532). Others, like Begun (1985), have cited the more general economic, regulatory, and societal shifts that were described in Chapters Two through Four as moving physicians and health care management into more conflictual roles.

Several assumptions about conflict between physicians and managers underlie the arguments we have included in this category. One is that physician and hospital interests in the pre-PPS period were aligned (Glandon & Morrisey, 1986). This implies that physician-manager relations in "the old days" used to be harmonious and that contextual shifts in the practice of medicine have undermined that harmony. Burns, Anderson and Shortell (1990) present a more complex view, arguing that although physician-manager relationships in the pre-PPS era were also conflictual, the conflict was amenable to management by compromise and avoidance. As medical practice moves into organizational settings such conflict resolution strategies ultimately become untenable: the more physicians practice within organizational settings, the more interdependent managers and doctors become. Key clinical and administrative issues in the delivery of services cannot be resolved if managers and doctors are not willing to confront their differences.

Another assumption in the contextual perspective is that the structural relationships of physician groups to health care organizations drives the quality of interactions among individual managers and physicians. Some research assesses the effectiveness of different institutional arrangements between physicians and hospitals (Begun, Luke, & Pointer, 1990; Stoeckle & Reiser, 1992). Other work categorizes and evaluates mechanisms, such as physician involvement on boards and restrictive admitting privileges, used to align physician behavior with institutional goals (Alexander & Morrisey, 1988; Burns, Andersen, & Shortell, 1989, 1990; Glandon & Morrisey, 1986; Smith, Reid, & Piland, 1990).

There is some disagreement in this research about what the contextual changes mean for the autonomy of physicians, and therefore about their impact on the nature and severity of manager-physician conflict. Have physicians inevitably become more like employees in a bureaucratic environment, or can certain structural arrangements guarantee that they can still practice as autonomous professionals? Much of the literature argues that this shift towards employee status is inevitable as managers are forced to respond to competitive and regulatory forces by developing mechanisms to control physician behavior. Others contend that physician autonomy can remain intact, within structural arrangements such as separate physician administrative hierarchies (Begun, Luke, & Pointer, 1990) or in the "loose coupling" of physicians to hospitals (Scott, 1982). Begun, Luke, and Pointer (1990) propose a model suggesting that a variety of structural linkages between physicians and health care organizations may be appropriate, depending on the nature of the competitive environment in which the organization operates.

It is noteworthy that while some articles treat the trend toward employment of physicians by organizations as an option consistent with the provision of good health care, other writers see it as detrimental to the practice of medicine, to the status of physicians, and to the mission of hospitals (Stoeckle & Reiser, 1992). In their analysis, contextual changes have shifted the power within health care organizations inappropriately and deleteriously toward administrators, thus causing the physician-manager dysfunction.

The dominant model of organizations and individuals in this analysis is economic. Managerial interests are assumed to be identical to organizational interests, which are assumed to be dominated by such economic concerns as costs, prices, and market share. Their preoccupation with these issues is assumed to be the primary reason managers would come into conflict with physicians: managers want to limit expenditures, and that necessarily compromises physician autonomy. Physician behavior is assumed to be sensitive to incentives and other control structures. Based on these assumptions, the management strategies suggested in this body of work are to assess organizational structures and incentives and to identify those that produce physician behavior most congruent with an organization's interests. Unfortunately, some research suggests that these incentive- and control-oriented strategies do not reliably produce desirable (or even expected) behavioral outcomes.

## The Professional Perspective

Much of the literature on health care administration and on medical practice in general takes note of the strong professional culture that shapes physicians' expectations and drives their behavior. This perspective assumes that the trouble in physician-manager relationships springs from a source other than contextual changes. Instead, the professional perspective considers physician-manager relations in health care organizations to be a manifestation of the familiar dynamics experienced in a variety of settings (for example, law firms, investment banks, universities, and high-tech firms) in which the people to be managed are professionals. Professionals devalue managers and management activities, preferring instead to concentrate entirely on their professional work, which they consider important, challenging, and gratifying. Managers tend to see professionals as uncooperative prima donnas who prefer to remain ignorant about the *real* business of the business they practice.

What we are calling the professional perspective stems from a well-established sociological tradition that characterizes the nature of professions and professional work (Abbott, 1988) and the difficulty that managers (as one category of employee) experience in working with professionals (as another category) in organizational settings (Benson, 1973; Satow, 1975). Raelin (1985) argues that managers and professionals are fundamentally different in their socialization and organizational roles and so inevitably come into conflict. Areas of conflict cited between professionals and managers include the professional's resistance to bureaucratic rules, rejection of bureaucratic standards, resistance to supervision, and conditional loyalty to the organization (Scott, 1966).

Although sociologists have examined the profession of medicine in some detail, the professional perspective appears in the health care literature as a largely unexplored assertion: the professionalization of doctors is likely to be mentioned as one of several factors inevitably complicating the efforts of health care managers to influence physicians. This perspective can be found in analyses of the impact of the physician's professional culture on the functioning of health care organizations (Fried, 1989), changes in the professional status of physicians (Freidson, 1985), and the role that socialization into the profession plays in shaping physician behavior (Krantz, 1984).

This perspective would suggest that, as dramatic as recent changes in the environment have been for the health care industry, tensions between physicians and managers are nothing new. The contextual changes have merely intensified them: "On one level, greater resource scarcity and competition for resources puts a greater emphasis on the *management* [emphasis ours] of professionals. On another, the changing character of work organizations (i.e., the breaking down of hierarchical controls, the need for collaborative structures) is in direct conflict with the idea of (professional) autonomy" (Krantz, 1984, p. 43).

Freidson (1985) takes this argument one step further, also linking professional-manager relationships to context. Researchers should look at the medical profession itself as an organization, he says. If the profession is well organized and funded, it may even be able to influence some of the contextual changes themselves—for example, legislated health care reform—through the actions of powerful groups such as the American Medical Association (AMA).

This thinking suggests that specific organizational factors have little bearing on the problem and that clashes will occur *whatever* the setting. Several older studies, however, identified factors that appear to mitigate conflict between managers and professionals: one is that older and longer-tenured professionals tend to be more accommodating in organizational settings (Abrahamson, 1964; Raelin, 1985). The potential for such conflict also appears to increase as the size of the organization increases (Abrahamson, 1964) and to decrease with the presence of professionals acting in managerial roles (Goss, 1961). Unfortunately, we could find no empirical work written from the professional perspective that brings these results up to date.

To fully explore this perspective, we must also point out that one can use the term *professional* to refer to managers as well as doctors. Physician-manager conflict can reasonably be seen as a clash of two specific professional cultures (Raelin, 1985) rather than as a conflict between a technician manager and a professional doctor. Descriptions of the two professional cultures support this view.

The medical profession is described as tightly bounded and highly socialized, commanding a loyalty from members that surpasses their loyalty to employing organizations (Freidson, 1985). The profession tends to take unilateral stands in support of its interests and to have significant clout via the AMA and other organizations in relevant public policy arenas. Highly internalized practice standards and well-articulated codes of ethics guide physician behavior, adherence to which is enforced (with debatable efficacy, however) by the organized profession.

In a more limited way, social science writers have also described management as a profession because of the ways managers are socialized to take characteristic approaches to problem-solving (Schön, 1983; Senge, 1990). Although recent revisions of MBA curricula across the country have provoked debate about how managers should be trained and socialized (Boyatzis, Cowen, Kolb, & Associates, 1994), the extension of this debate into the health care arena is little in evidence.

Few studies have been designed to explore whether or not disputes between physicians and managers are primarily the expression of conflict between two professions, medicine and management. Interestingly, much of the writing about professionals, like that reviewed as representing the contextual perspective, assumes that physician behavior, shaped by professional socialization and cultural norms, not manager behavior, is the primary cause of difficulties between the two groups.

However the argument is formulated, the concept of power that appears so prominently in the contextual work runs through this literature as well. Will physicians continue to "control" the delivery of health care, or is the "dominance" of their profession waning as the "power" of the professional manager rises (Freidson, 1985; Coburn, 1992)? This is essentially a sociological argument focusing on the power of physicians as a class relative to the power of managers.

Conflict resolution strategies developed from this perspective might take several forms: balancing the professional power of physicians and managers through strategies that emphasize the importance of both to the organization; strengthening health care managers' professional organizations so they can compete more effectively with physician organizations; devising schemes to balance physician loyalty to the medical profession by increasing their identification with the health care organizations in which they work; and overcoming destructive stereotypes by raising physician and manager consciousness of the often undiscussed assumptions and values that guide behaviors in the "other" professional culture. One widely adopted tactic in this category is the increasing use of physicians themselves in managerial roles.

## The Organizational Perspective

A third perspective reflected in the research on physician-manager relations focuses on health care organizations themselves. One view is that the organizations simply cannot be managed because they are so complex and because physician-manager difficulties are so intractable. Another is that though the job is difficult it is doable, but current administrators lack the skills and competencies necessary to meet the challenge.

Interestingly, this perspective appears to shift the responsibility for tensions in the relationship away from physicians exclusively. The focus is instead on the kinds of work done in health care organizations, how that work is and must be organized, and how well managers are prepared to run these complex systems. Like the contextual perspective, this view focuses on structures. But instead of blaming changes in the external environment for the conflict, the organizational view examines the nature of the work done *inside* the organization and the administrative structures required to get it done.

The organizational view also offers different assumptions about the universality of manager-physician conflict. The contextual or professional views assume that primary causality for conflict lies outside the boundaries of health care organizations and that therefore managerial solutions at the organization level may be difficult to find. Instead, the organizational view implies that, in theory, organization-specific solutions to conflict are available, though perhaps not easily accessible, through the behavior of people inside the organization in the form of better management processes and systems.

This perspective raises fundamental questions about the extent to which health care organizations are essentially similar to or different from other complex organizations and, more specifically, other organizations in which managers work with professionals. The debate in the literature seems to rest on such questions as: How different are they? Is the management profession competent enough to understand those differences as they import models from other sectors into health care settings?

Most of the articles in this stream take a sober, if not pessimistic, view (Weisbord, 1976). Many writers, not just those cited here, make reference to the structural dilemma in health care organizations represented in Scott's paper (1982): the dual administrative and clinical authority ladders that intersect only at the top. Begun (1985) and Stoelwinder (1982), for example, describe the urgency of coordination across these two systems but stress the continued obstacles to management presented by the physicians' professional assertion of the prerogative to control clinical work. Here, the intent is not to paint the culture of the medical profession as unreasonable, but rather to describe a fundamental "flaw" or core managerial puzzle inherent in health care organizations: managers are responsible for their organizations' continued viability without being in charge of the core organizational task, patient care.

Weisbord's much-quoted 1976 article makes this point by discussing the intractability of health care organizations to traditional consultative and management improvement techniques. He describes a structural problem that is more complex than the dual hierarchy model would suggest, one without easy solution. The missing links in his scheme are between three systems that are integrated in a typical industrial environment: task (how the primary work gets done in the various key categories—patient care, research, education, and so on), identity (how professionals develop and move through career paths and therefore how they are motivated), and governance (how standards are set for performance and how behaviors are measured against those standards). Weisbord argued that at the time he was writing health care managers faced an impossible situation: they had no leverage over the identity system and little leverage over the task system, yet they were ultimately responsible for the performance and viability of the organization. Given the environmental changes that have occurred in recent years, today's managers may have more leverage, but since physicians remain the experts on whom the organization depends to deliver its primary service, the physicians retain some leverage of their own.

Other writers suggest that the fundamental and problematic "difference" in health care organizations is located as much in the nature of the work as in the structure. Shortell and Kaluzny (1983) list some characteristics of the work done in health care organizations. For example, they describe the work as highly variable and complex, and often done on an emergency basis. There is little tolerance for error in this work, and not infrequently the activities require close coordination among diverse professional groups (pp. 13–14). Raising questions about just *how* different health care organizations are, the authors agree that "health care organizations may be unusual if not unique in that many of them possess all of the above characteristics *in combination* [emphasis theirs]" (p. 14).

However, Shortell and Kaluzny stop short of the next step taken by other writers, who argue that it is the *emotional* dimension of health care work that makes these organizations both unique and extremely difficult to manage. Merrill and Moosbruker (1982) characterize hospitals as the settings in which societal fears about illness are acted out. In hospitals, patients become low-status outcasts, and physicians are expected to be priests or magicians. Krantz (1984), representing a sociotechnical perspective in which the social and technical aspects of work are recognized as inextricably linked, argues that the emotions generated by such notions of illness and clinical treatment (dependency, grandiosity, anxiety, denial) have a strong impact on how work is organized in health care settings. As demonstrated by Menzies (1975) in her classic study of nurses, administrative systems seem designed as much to assist clinicians in managing their own strong and difficult emotional reactions to their work as to assure the most efficient and effective treatment. Many of the stories recounted by Heymann (1995) can be explained in the same way.

Fried questioned whether these emotional dynamics impact the applicability of organizational theory to the health care environment: "While theory proposes to cut across organizational types, the question arises as to whether health services organizations are sufficiently distinct from other organizations to require different ways of viewing and measuring organizational phenomena. Specifically, two ubiquitous characteristics of health services organizations may confound the application of theories of organization: the life and death environment . . . and the presence of physicians" who, his research shows, "confound theory about how groups gain power in institutional settings" (Fried, 1989, p. 925).

Several writers in the organizational development (OD) field present a variation on this organizational view that is uncharacteristically judgmental about managerial performance. For example, Cummings and Huse (1989) and Nadler and Tichy (1982) are among the most prominent writers who argue that planned change efforts do not work well in health care settings because health care managers are not up to the job: they simply do not have the skills to handle these complex organizations. Munson and Zuckerman (1983) offer a more detailed explanation: health care managers focus too much on financial management and not enough on organizational issues such as reward systems, leadership, and decision making.

In arguing that OD work in health care organizations should focus primarily on structural problems, Plovnik (1982) also touches on questions about the crisis-oriented nature of the work and the absence of managerial acumen. In his formulation, OD consultants can provide the kind of structural expertise that health care managers lack. Explanations for the absence of managerial competence in health care settings, however, are not provided.

Not surprisingly, the organizational view is influenced by the fields of organizational behavior and organizational development. The assumption embedded in these fields is that organizations *can* be managed well; therefore, if they are not, one should look at the fit between internal management systems and the nature of the work done in the organization. From this perspective, the presence of professional physicians is probably not by itself the root cause of managerial problems because managers in other settings seem to have learned how to manage professionals. Thus, the problem must be located specifically inside health care organizations as a category of organization and traced to their structure, to the nature of the organizational tasks, to managerial competence, or to all of the above.

Interestingly, the belief in the efficacy of management that lies behind this view takes physicians off the hook: the organizations themselves, or at least the managers who run them, are seen as the primary source of the problem. Conflict resolution strategies could include creating better structural mechanisms to link clinical and administrative tasks, developing clear remedies for dysfunctional systemic accommodations to the emotional difficulty of health care work, and devoting more resources to recruiting and training the best managers for health care organizations.

## The Intergroup Perspective

Intergroup theorists in organizational behavior suggest that the inevitably differing perspectives and priorities of functional groups *within organizations* bring them naturally into conflict (Bettner & Collins, 1987). The more divergent the groups' perspectives (based on the nature of the work they do, the reward systems for each group, and the history of relations between the groups), the greater the conflict.

In most health care organizations, for example, much of the work physicians do is crisis-oriented, highly specialized, individually focused work caring for patients, while managers tend to work on more abstract, longer-term problems related to securing or maintaining viability for the institution. Physicians focus on micro-level questions of patient health and managers on macro-level issues of utilization patterns, efficiency, and quality (see Scott, 1982). Physicians are concerned with having access to the resources they need to do their jobs; managers focus on controlling the use of those resources. Thus, the two groups have different jobs, which give them different perspectives and bring them into conflict about a variety of organizational policies, practices, and values. Such tensions can be understood as resembling the familiar intraorganizational functional conflict in business among research and development, manufacturing, marketing, and sales departments.

This view is similar to the professional perspective discussed earlier, but it focuses on group differences *within* organizations. From the intergroup perspective, specific physician-manager conflict in organization X is more a product of conditions among groups in organization X than of the extraorganizational professional training or socialization of physicians or managers. In this formulation, professional identity may intensify differences between organizational groups, but the severity and character of the conflict can vary in different organizations, depending on the history of relations between the groups, on the structure of the groups' work, on the culture of the specific organization, and even on the presence of particular individuals in key positions (charismatic leaders or diplomats or autocrats).

This perspective also has similarities to the organizational one because it is looking inside the organization, but it differs in an important way. In the organizational perspective the focus is on the organization as a whole, its structures and tasks. The intergroup focus is on the work of specific groups *within* an organization, on the ways physicians and managers in different units and at different hierarchical levels do or do not coordinate and communicate with each other, on the relative influence of each group, and on the historical dynamics of the intergroup relationship inside the organization.

In a special 1978 issue of the *Journal of Applied Behavioral Science* devoted to health care systems, Weisbord and Goodstein reflected: "There have been very few efforts to study entire systems—that is, the relationships among physicians and nurses, for example, or physicians, administrators, nurses and technicians in the delivery of care" (1978, p. 264). Since then, there seems to be far more intergroup research examining physician-nurse relationships in health care organizations than relations between physicians and managers.

Alt-White, Charns, and Strayer (1983) did look more directly at intergroup relations, but they omitted administrators. They discovered the strongest predictors of nurse-physician collaboration were a work design that required nurses, like physicians, to focus on specific patients, and managerial norms that fostered open communication and positive working climates.

In the OD tradition, many writers (Delbecq & Gill, 1985; Lammert, 1978; Stoelwinder & Clayton, 1978) have taken an intergroup perspective in describing efforts to create teams mixing groups of clinical professionals. However, administrators have consistently been left out of this intergroup picture! One article moves toward the administrative arena in considering the nurse's role in linking clinical and administrative dimensions of patient care (Merrill & Moosbruker, 1982); however, administrators themselves are omitted.

We found only two articles that looked empirically at physician-manager conflict. Weisbord, Lawrence, and Charns (1978) identified modes of conflict resolution employed across the physician-manager boundary as well as among medical school departments. However, this was only one dimension of a much larger study focusing on a wide variety of management issues in academic teaching hospitals. Bettner and Collins (1987) appear to base their analysis of the phases of physician-manager conflict on empirical information, but they do not identify the sources of their data. (While Fried, 1989, examined power acquisition of physicians, nurses, and administrators, his research did not explore the relationships among these groups.)

The intergroup view, like the organizational, is grounded in the organizational behavior and organizational development areas, but it focuses more on behavior (group dynamics, interpersonal interactions) than on organizational structures and systems. This perspective leaves room for specific solutions in organizational units or departments that would open boundaries across groups to increase cooperation. Some of these "solutions" can already be found in certain health care environments: utilizing in key roles the person who can see both sides (the physician acting in a managerial role), initiating face-to-face meetings between physician and manager groups, and creating joint leadership structures for certain departments of medical and nonmedical managers.

## The Individual Perspective

The final perspective we explore here locates the conflict between managers and physicians primarily in their *individual* differences. Despite the absence of empirical work from this perspective, one could argue that this is the dominant "theory-in-use" among health care providers, managers, and consumers. People seem to act *as if* it is true. Administrators may recognize that doctors are socialized to carry certain attitudes, but they still are likely to attribute physician behavior to personality traits (arrogance, lack of empathy, selfishness) rather than to organizational role or group membership.

This view offers an explanation for the conflict in the assumption that doctors and managers have predictable, and profoundly different, personality types. If it were to be developed explicitly, the argument would rest on personality theory as it relates to occupational choice and careers (Holland, 1973), individual learning styles (Wolfe & Kolb, 1984), and cognitive characteristics (Frese, 1982), and also on theories of interpersonal relations, for example, conflict resolution (Deutsch, 1973) and communication styles (Bowen, 1982; Rogers & Farson, 1976).

The line of thought can be summarized as follows, taking the stereotypical view of the physician first. Certain kinds of people are more likely than others to choose the medical profession and to survive medical school training. They are competitive, technically oriented, eager to specialize, and ready to sacrifice significantly in the short-term for a long-term career payoff in money, social status, and intellectual challenge. They choose the doctor mythology for their primary personal identity. This perspective also assumes that people select medical specialties because of characteristic personality factors; it would say, for example, that strong-willed, intolerant, technically oriented people become surgeons, while gentler, easygoing people become pediatricians.

This perspective poses an explanation for the tensions between managers and physicians that is different from that offered by the professional view. From the individual vantage point, the culture of the profession is shaped and reinforced by the personalities of the practitioners. For example, arguably in order to accommodate the personality-determined preferences of physicians to control their own environment, the medical profession has relied on peer supervision to monitor quality. However, since peers have been reluctant to criticize each others' work because they share the same traits, this perspective asserts that physician misconduct is often unreported or too easily forgiven.

This "personality hypothesis" can also be used to explain why physicians working in organizational environments may be dissatisfied and stressed (Carton, 1995). Because physicians value autonomy and historically have practiced under conditions that reinforced that attitude, they feel frustrated working within the confines of institutional constraints. From this perspective, the reluctance to delimit one's own and others' autonomy can be seen as a personality trait, as much as a product of professional socialization.

A similar stereotypical picture can be drawn of the manager: controlling, data-driven, procedure-oriented, penny-pinching. A number of personality or learning-style inventories consistently identify a "managerial" type, distinct from the personality type or style associated with other professions. For example, managers have been identified as individuals who generally prefer concrete experience and active experimentation as learning modes over abstract conceptualization and reflective observation (Wolfe & Kolb, 1984).

Depending on the nature of the attributes associated with each personality, the primary blame for physician-manager conflict can be placed on either side: managers have an impossible task because doctors are unmanageable by disposition, or physicians have to fight to practice good medicine in the face of bureaucratic pencil-pushers who want control for the sake of control.

Although this individual perspective is quite prominent in the writing on health care, there is little research that tests the argument. For example, the characterization of managers as "accommodating" types who are best at doing things, taking risks, and encountering new experiences has not been tested on health care managers. Nor does it even fit the picture, sometimes seen in the literature, of health care managers as "agents of bureaucracy."

So far as we know, no one has even employed the Myers-Briggs Type Indicator (MBTI), the widely used personality inventory, to test if physicians disproportionately fall into one or another of the sixteen possible profiles (Hirsh & Kummerow, 1990). According to a career-choice book based on the MBTI, physicians tend to be introverted (oriented more to their inner world than to the world outside) and thinking (making decisions logically rather than emotionally) types (Tieger & Barron-Tieger, 1992). However, no empirical work testing physicians and managers is reported. In fact, this same book suggests that the two groups of professionals *share* some of these same traits.

Kurtz (1994) did establish empirically that by temperament physicians have a high need for power, control, and dominance and need to be the focal point in decision structures. However, the implications of this personality type compared with different managerial temperaments, if any can be identified, have not been explored.

Managerial strategies that would be based on this theoretical perspective are remarkably like those that *are* employed to manage physicians. For example, an advocate of this view might counsel conflict avoidance first, on the theory that conflict is rooted in personality and people's personalities cannot be changed. Approaches to conflict resolution (given that conflict is *un*avoidable) might include looking for the "few" physicians and managers with atypical personality types to serve in key liaison positions, avoiding meetings and other processes that might invoke interpersonal confrontation, and employing a "need-to-know" strategy for managing information. The general approach would be to leave well enough alone, but when conflict erupts, to employ bargaining to settle physician-manager disputes (Weisbord, Lawrence, & Charns,

1978). This in a nutshell appears to be the management strategy most commonly reported by observers of health care organizations (Kralewski, 1995). We believe that, given the increasing complexity of medical care processes, this approach will increasingly be inadequate to the challenges faced by health care organizations in the late 1990s and beyond.

## Conclusions

We have examined these five perspectives separately to simplify and organize our discussion of existing work on physician-manager relationships. However, in treating these views separately, we want to be careful not to perpetuate the view that they are mutually exclusive. We do not believe that one perspective can or will eventually be proven "correct" at the expense of others. Each of these five perspectives contains useful truths, and none should be dismissed. Each captures an important dimension of a complex problem: individual, organizational, and environmental factors *do* affect physician-manager relations. We present them separately for their heuristic value in helping readers recognize that multiple perspectives exist, reflecting fundamentally different analyses of the causes of a very complex set of relationships. The solution to the problem of dysfunctional physician-manager relations clearly lies in the integration of these views.

Another risk in the discussion presented here is that it may give the false impression that these perspectives have carried equal weight thus far in the writing and thinking about health care. In fact, most of the writing we examined was rooted in the contextual and professional perspectives. Not much empirical work has been done to reflect the intergroup and individual viewpoints, and most of the organizational work is twenty years old. We believe that the unequal weight of attention to the various disciplinary perspectives has had important implications for the health care field, both in the effort to build an effective research agenda and in the search for practical ways of producing more effective physician-manager relations for the 1990s and beyond.

Thus, both problems—the lack of integration across perspectives and the imbalance in the research conducted so far—must be addressed if progress is to be made. We offer next some thoughts about how this might be accomplished, in the academic as well as the practical arenas.

## Research

First, some research methodologies have been employed much more extensively than others. To expand our general understanding of this issue, the range of methodologies must be extended beyond the survey techniques that are most frequently mobilized in studies from the contextual and professional perspectives. Some social science fields view survey responses as limited in value because they do not capture important differences across organizations and because they reflect attitudes and reported rather than real behaviors. While our view is that surveys and the sophisticated statistical methods associated with them have enormous value, research reflecting the organizational, intergroup, and individual orientations can benefit from time-intensive immersion in organizations to understand the specific structures, histories, and cultures of particular institutions and the roles they play in influencing the behavior of individual physicians and managers. From this perspective, face-to-face interviews and observation, analyzed using appropriate qualitative techniques, are valuable tools of data collection that at the very least can enrich the interpretation of survey results by creating a clear, three-dimensional picture of the critical organizational context.

Electing a more inclusive approach that includes field research does not require throwing out or devaluing the work already published on physician-manager relations. However, it does mean initiating efforts to link prior results to new empirical work that focuses on the understudied intraorganizational parts of the puzzle. This linking work within individual projects and across a number of studies requires the willingness and ability of researchers (as well as evaluators, consumers, and sponsors of the research) to think across disciplinary boundaries.

From this perspective, a research agenda is more than a series of studies focusing on previously underresearched areas. That kind of piecemeal approach may help flesh out different parts of the puzzle of physician-manager relationships, but it does not build a comprehensive picture of a complex organizational problem influenced by a multiplicity of factors both external and internal to the organization. A research agenda in this new sense means bringing together ideas from different traditions in the planning and execution of new studies. It means helping researchers learn to consider the implications of the work of their colleagues and competitors from other backgrounds and disciplines.

## Real-World Solutions

On a more pragmatic level, the imbalance among the variety of perspectives reflected in the academic literature and the lack of integrative thinking across disciplines may also have constrained efforts to solve real problems in physician-manager relationships. Managerial training, of course, is largely conducted in academic settings and likely to be influenced by instructors' disciplinary training. Whether health care curricula are dominated by "economic" rather than "organizational" perspectives, or vice versa, a curriculum focused on teaching separate functions (for example, accounting, finance, operations, organizational behavior, marketing) without attending to integration among them will not help the next generation of health care managers. The ability to create specific structures and systems to integrate clinical and administrative functions is the skill they will need most.

Also, we have argued that independent of what is found in the professional or academic literature, managers and physicians often seem to operate intuitively out of certain conceptual models—especially the individual personality model. In the absence of close, explicit testing of that "theory," health care professionals may never be forced to reexamine their prejudices and new solutions may not be applied throughout the field.

In our view, the goal for health care researchers should be to integrate the insights from each of the five perspectives into a unified model of physician-manager relations, which can account for different solutions for different groups and organizations that operate in different times and markets. In the next chapter we present one approach to generating such a theory, which we hope will prove useful as a guide for future research projects.

For managers, the goal is to find intervention points and design strategies that can result in improvements in an organization's performance. Those more narrowly targeted actions may in fact derive from analysis based on one of the five perspectives. However, even for very practically oriented managers, integrated theory has value in helping them keep the big picture both in their own minds and in front of physicians. Every policy they put into place has impacts (some unintended) on the wider organization. Theory should be useful to these managers in anticipating the impact of the decisions they make to improve physician-manager relations. In Chapter Nine we explore the implications of a more integrative approach for both doctors and managers.

# 8

# An Open Systems View

## A Realistic Framework for the Health Care Organization

Managers and physicians must learn to work together more effectively, and we believe they can. The first step is for managers to learn to bring a new, more comprehensive perspective to defining and solving problems. The factors that influence physicians and managers in health care settings are complex and inextricably linked to other problems facing the organization. To bring about change, managers must move beyond focusing on narrowly defined problem "solutions" (for example, compensation arrangements based on the assumption that clinical decisions are determined by the financial incentives physicians face) to working on a wider range of organizational fronts. This more inclusive approach reflects an understanding that behavior has multiple determinants and that activities in an organization are interrelated.

While specific suggestions to improve relations are likely to come from physicians and managers on the front lines who have learned how to collaborate, organizational theory has much to contribute to this discussion. In this chapter, we present a realistic model of the health care organization *as the context* in which physician-manager problem solving must occur. This model can help the two groups develop a broader perspective on the issues affecting their collaboration and a sharper picture of what needs to change.

As a first step, we lay out an integrative framework building on the five perspectives discussed in Chapter Seven. This model for organizations is called an *open systems view* and is the source of the depiction of the five perspectives shown in Figure 7.1. In the first part of this chapter, we explore connections among the perspectives and argue that the open systems framework is a useful aid for analyzing performance problems in health care organizations. Later, we return to the stories of Chapter One to illustrate the diagnostic value of the framework in understanding breakdowns in physician-manager relations. Then, in the final chapter, we move forward to suggest specific means for clarifying and strengthening physician-manager relations in specific health care organizations. In that chapter, we show how open systems theory points managers to the tools they need to create organizational conditions in which both they and their physician colleagues can practice with increased satisfaction.

## The Health Care Organization as an Open System

The open systems framework is a theoretical view of organizations that underlies much of the management and organizational literature, although as noted at the end of the previous chapter, it has not been fully exploited as a guide to empirical research on physician-manager relations. A particular strength of the open systems framework is that it captures the complex interdependencies between organizations and their environments, as well as among various internal elements of each organization. The model helps explain the importance of both structural and behavioral perspectives on organizations. As a result, it can inform both "hard" management decisions (restructuring, implementation of new information systems) as well as initiatives on the "soft" side (practices to improve the processes of care, relations between groups, or patient satisfaction).

The power of the open systems model derives in part from the assumption that while organizations in the same industry have some common features, each is also different from the others. Each adapts differently to its environment and achieves a unique, more or less successful balance among competing internal needs for resources.

The model makes clear that there can be no single formula for success for an organization and therefore no cookbook of strategies for managers to follow. Each manager must analyze the particular situation he or she faces, devise and implement a strategy, and then, again with the help of the open systems framework, analyze the responses to the strategy and adapt to still newer conditions that continue to emerge. Many roads can lead to positive outcomes; conversely, many decisions can derail an organization's progress toward desired results.

The model recognizes that the internal units of an organization are often engaged in enterprises quite different from one another. Thus, structures and/or policies that work well in one unit may not foster the desired level of productive activity in another with which it interacts. For example, a primary care group that streamlines its operations may not be providing enough information about the patients it refers to a specialty department in order for the specialists to serve them well. Similarly, in developing its own procedures, that specialty group may not pay enough attention to maximizing the value of the tests and other work performed by their primary care colleagues. The result can be duplication and waste for the MCO as a whole and poor service to its patients. The vignette "Uncoordinated Care" in Chapter Six, which presents the case of a cardiac patient, illustrates the problem.

The model also makes clear that an organization cannot function as a loose federation of units acting independently of each other. There must be enough centralization of decision making and coordination among units to ensure effective outcomes and efficient use of resources. At the most basic level, coordination is essential to prevent the organization from falling into chaos. Too much centralization, however, will stifle innovation and limit the organization's ability to adapt to new circumstances.

The contextual and professional perspectives presented in Chapter Seven are concerned mainly with the impact of macro-level, large-scale, generic environmental forces on a whole population of similar organizations and do not account for the impact of environmental changes on *specific* organizations. Nor do they allow us to explain in detail why some organizations adapt well to the changes while others adapt poorly. The field can benefit, therefore, from a framework that allows more careful observation of specific organizations' efforts to adapt to those critical external pressures.

In the discussion that follows, we describe the open systems model in more detail and then explain how it can be used to build an integrative view of the forces influencing physician-manager relations in health care organizations.

## The Open Systems Model

A system is defined as an entity consisting of interacting and mutually interdependent subunits. Its viability depends on the effective interaction of the components, or subsystems, to create a coherent whole (Cummings & Huse, 1989). The subsystems in organizations are, for example, the different divisions, units, and hierarchical levels that interact to keep the organization viable.

Open systems are distinguished from closed systems in that they are influenced to a significant degree by (are "open" to) forces from outside the system itself. Hospitals, for example, are influenced by state regulations establishing conditions for licenses to operate, by policies of insurance companies that set rules for receiving payments, and by the actions of competing organizations that are trying to lure away physicians and patients. Thus, organizations conceptualized as open systems are characterized by another structural feature: physical, symbolic, and/or behavioral mechanisms that form a boundary differentiating the organization from the environment that surrounds it. Open systems, like human organizations, rely for survival on a regular exchange of information and other resources across the boundary with their environment (Morgan, 1986).

### Origins

The open systems model stems from Von Bertalanffy's (1968) attempt to devise a "general systems" theory to explain all levels of life activity in humans, from biological activity at the intracellular level to political and economic activity at the societal level. Social scientists at the Tavistock Clinic in England (for example, Emery & Trist, 1965; Miller & Rice, 1967) refined this work to develop a set of open systems concepts that helped explain group and organizational dynamics.

Since then, social scientists in a variety of disciplines have continued to refine the application of the open systems model to human systems of various scales. Professionals in each discipline have applied the model to the levels of analysis that traditionally have distinguished their own field from those of others: sociologists have applied it to societal groups such as social classes or ethnicities in their research on power relations among large social groups; organizational behaviorists have applied it to organizations in their study of coordination and control among organizational units; group and family psychologists have applied it to human groups in explaining dynamics among family members and work groups; and psychologists have applied it to the individual in considering, for example, how individuals become psychologically differentiated from one another. These are the same "levels" of analysis, proceeding from the societal down to the individual, that are represented in the five perspectives of Chapter Seven.

## Core Principles

The five key concepts in open systems theory—structure, throughput, boundaries, integration, and homeostasis—are discussed in the following paragraphs. Each concept helps to clarify the management dilemmas typical of health care organizations.

### Structure: Hierarchy of Levels/Differentiation

Open systems are assumed to be structured in hierarchical fashion, with smaller systems embedded in larger ones. Organizations, for example, are composed of groups, which in turn are composed of individuals. The organization itself, from this perspective, represents one hierarchical level in a still larger human social system—say, the health care industry—which may itself be a subsystem of several larger systems (the nation). Figure 7.1 shows this embedded structure, with the organization as the middle level. Through this lens, physicians and managers can be seen as members of *both* larger, extraorganizational social units, including their professions, and smaller groups within their organizations. Their behavior is influenced to a greater or lesser extent by all of these memberships.

The structure of open systems such as organizations is still more complex than this description might suggest, however. Even subunits within the organization are differentiated by function, and individuals in an organization are typically members of several different subunits at the same time. For example, physicians in a hospital are members of a large organizational subunit defined by profession. They have specialized credentials and are expected to perform tasks and roles that are differentiated from the tasks performed by members of other groups (lab technicians, nurses, cafeteria workers). At the same time, however, a physician practicing in an outpatient clinic at the hospital shares subunit membership with the nurses, social workers, dieticians, administrators, and other individuals who work in the clinic. The clinic *also* represents a specialized function within the organization, one to which a variety of different kinds of professionals contribute.

Thus, open systems are differentiated into specialized subunits, and individuals experience complex and overlapping group memberships *within* health care organizations.

### Throughput

From cells to organizations, open systems require processes called *throughput* for survival. Resources (inputs) are taken into the system from the environment, transformed (throughput), and then sent back out to the environment (outputs). For example, a hospital takes in medical technology, equipment, personnel, and patients. The staff utilizes the equipment and technology to treat the patients, who are then discharged to the environment in a condition different from their state when they entered (for example, recovered from an illness). Information about this experience is another product of the process which, when fed back into the system, influences subsequent transformation processes.

The concept suggests that both physicians and managers are actors in the throughput process, but with differentiated roles. Among other things, managers acquire the equipment and take responsibility for establishing the procedures that result in a patient's expeditious movement through the system (from appointment-setting to visit with a clinician to lab tests to treatment). Physicians, along with other clinicians, provide the medical care that brought the patient to the hospital. In the throughput process, the managerial and physician roles are not only interrelated but also interdependent.

If the managers do not establish a well-operating appointment process that gets patients to the hospital when they require care and when doctors can see them, then the organization wastes resources. Similarly, if a patient and physician are in an examining room together but the physician does not have the medical records or supplies he needs to perform the necessary services, that too is wasteful.

Thus, for a health care organization to function efficiently, managers and physicians must each contribute in a coordinated fashion to the throughput process, so that the required tasks can be performed effectively using as few resources as possible. The concept of throughput makes clear the essential interdependencies among various system members.

## Boundaries

When applied to organizations, "boundary" is an abstraction, but the concept is analogous to the permeable and visible wall that regulates throughput in living cells, for example. In human systems, the term *boundary* refers to the managerial and psychological *processes* that distinguish system units from one another and the system as a whole from its environment. Organizational transactions with the environment (for example, intake or discharge procedures), as well as transactions among subsystems inside the organization, are regulated by boundaries, which vary in degree of permeability.

Regulating the flow of patients into, through, and out of the organization (such as a hospital inpatient subsystem) is crucial to system effectiveness. If too few patients come in (if the boundary is too hard to permeate), the hospital's capacity is underutilized. This might happen if the intake process is so cumbersome that patients— or physicians responding to their complaints—are discouraged from continuing to seek admission there and try other hospitals instead. It can also occur when payers, such as MCOs, make it harder for subscribers to obtain approval for an admission (they raise the barrier to admission in order to limit their own expenditures). In the first instance, the hospital may be able to increase admissions by streamlining its processes. If the second condition persists, however, it will have excess capacity, which will drain resources unless it can be transformed to other productive uses or at least be taken out of service to stop the loss.

Boundary permeability also plays a role at the other end of the caregiving process. For example, hospitals increasingly are discharging patients after shorter and shorter stays, primarily as a response to payer pressure. If organizational practices create boundaries that are too permeable, patients are discharged before they are sufficiently recovered, and their health can deteriorate as a result. Occupancy rate, the common measure showing the relationship between the organization's capacity and the demand for its services, is regulated in part by adjustments in the permeability of the hospital's boundary. Whether the reasons are under the hospital's control or not, it must adapt in order to thrive.

Another example of the key boundary-regulation function can be found in the flows of information about patients among units *within* a managed care organization. Those flows may be open or constrained, depending on how the system is organized and managed. For example, if a central information system connects all the clinical units in which a patient may be seen, a referring primary care physician can record information about the patient's history, and a specialist at another location can access and review it before the patient arrives. In order for that transfer to occur, the sites need not only the appropriate hardware and software but also routine procedures that lead the referring physician to enter the data and the specialist to access and use it. The vignette "Uncoordinated Care" in Chapter Six illustrates some of the consequences for a cardiac patient of failing to provide information across boundaries in a timely manner. While the smooth flow of information across subsystem boundaries is desirable, a balance must also be struck with the need for confidentiality, providing appropriate protections for sensitive patient information.

These examples illustrate ways in which physicians and managers share responsibility for boundary regulation. Physicians must see that their patients can get into the hospital when they need care and are discharged only as appropriate to their condition. They also must be sure that optimally useful information about their patients is transferred in a timely manner to the people who need it inside or outside the organization. At the organizational level, managers are responsible for setting up the administrative systems to ensure that capacity utilization is optimal and that information flow is timely and accurate. If these administrative processes break down or do not function well, then essential clinical work may be undermined.

### Integration

Systems typically consist of subsystems that are differentiated to perform certain essential specialized tasks. The entire system's efficient and effective functioning depends on coordination among those subunits. Although systems typically spend some of their resources to perform this integration function, breakdowns occur (again, as in the failure to transfer key patient information in the cardiac case).

One of the well-documented problems of health care management, for example, has been the lack of integration between financial information systems and clinical systems. In the past, this has prevented physicians from recognizing when their expenditures for a patient were mounting beyond a reasonable target level. Newer information systems allow physicians to see the cost of each test they order as well as the total cost of treatment to date. Increasingly, physicians are expected to consider cost as a factor in treatment decisions. When managers provide integrating information systems, physicians can consider whether the cost of the test is worth the additional information they expect it to produce.

In open-systems terms, money is one of the resources (input) that a physician has available as she or he determines the appropriate diagnosis and treatment processes (throughput) intended to create satisfied and healthier patients (output). Use of this finite resource requires that priorities be set. An integrated information system can be the link that permits clinicians to make effective caregiving decisions in a health care environment in which many highly specialized but interdependent activities create competing demands for limited resources.

### Homeostasis

This term refers to a kind of steady-state or self-correcting status achieved by a system's structures and processes in the regulation of all its activities. Information on the costs and benefits of system activities is fed back into the system, which continually adjusts to what it learns. The balance that is struck represents one solution to the problem of how system resources may best be deployed so that at a minimum the system can survive. As the external environment changes, the system must alter its internal functioning to continue to thrive.

For example, ambulatory services were once seen as decidedly secondary activities in hospitals. At first, they were offered in order to provide a site for ongoing contact between patients and hospital doctors after an initial inpatient stay. Later, they were used as the locus of ongoing doctor-patient contacts and became a source of patients to feed inpatient activities. Most of the hospital's resources were focused on supporting its inpatient services. As forces in the health care environment have reduced the demand for inpatient services and rewarded hospitals for cost containment, most hospitals have rebalanced their resource utilization. Thus, operating rooms, physician and nursing time, and patient intake systems, for example, are now more likely than previously to be focused on revenue-producing activities occurring in outpatient facilities rather than in costlier inpatient settings.

## Using the Open Systems Framework to Link the Five Perspectives

Applying the open systems framework to health care organizations allows us to integrate insights from the five perspectives described in Chapter Seven. First, by assuming that organizations have complex relationships with their environments, the framework accommodates the contextual and professional perspectives. It goes beyond them, however, by recognizing explicitly that different organizations will adapt differently to the same extraorganizational forces. It invites us to look inside the organization to explore how professional differences are managed, for example, instead of assuming that those differences are *always and equally* problematic to similar organizations in the same industry. It also allows us to understand the possibility that professional tensions might be managed more effectively in some units than in others in a single organization. The open systems framework offers the potential that managers can, over time, *learn to manage* the impact of external forces.

The open systems approach, congruent with the contextual perspective, posits a direct connection between environmental forces and organizational arrangements. Thus, it allows us to trace the impact of, for example, regulatory changes on the inner workings of a particular organization. It also invites us to look for the impact of external forces in unexpected places in the organization. For example, we might see adjustments to Medicare's prospective payment system (PPS) and diagnosis related groups (DRGs) not just in the introduction of actions to contain costs but also in the unintended impacts of those adaptations on employee morale and patient satisfaction. Thus, the framework recognizes that in trying to solve one problem, managers may unwittingly create or aggravate others. The managerial remedy again lies in anticipating and moderating specific "ripple effects" that adjustments to external forces can have on *all* aspects of organizational activity, not just those that are deliberately targeted.

The open systems framework also is sophisticated enough to encompass the peculiar characteristics that differentiate health care organizations from other organizations, including the complex "dual hierarchy" structure (Harris, 1977), the massive amount of information that must be captured and managed, and the emotional intensity of the work. Each of these features is common to health care organizations yet also representative of broadly shared organizational characteristics of internal differentiation, integration, and boundary regulation. Physician-manager relations are only one of several interconnected and difficult management problems.

The open systems framework permits observers to view the pattern of relations between these groups not as an isolated "personnel issue" but rather as one of several mechanisms by which a particular organization achieves homeostasis. The approach also allows us to understand why patterns of seemingly dysfunctional behavior can persist in organizations over long periods of time. The open systems framework suggests that a persisting pattern of overt conflict or conflict avoidance among groups in an organization serves *some* function, for example, protecting the dominance of each group in its own primary sphere. Although that pattern may not represent the most efficient use of resources, it can be tolerated if competitive pressures from the environment do not require that waste be eliminated.

Finally, the open systems framework also lets us examine complex causal explanations for behavior *within* complex health care organizations. Specifically, the actions of physicians and managers can be assessed at multiple levels of analysis within the system (individual, intergroup) to gain analytic leverage on a problem.

The open systems perspective allows us to focus our attention on two crucial components of physician-manager relations: structures and behaviors. By *structures* we mean formal hierarchical relationships, functional differentiation (units organized by physician specialty, such as cardiology or rheumatology), and job/role definitions inside organizations, as well as the formal institutional arrangements among groups of organizations or groups of physicians and health care organizations. By *behaviors* we mean the patterned, predictable interactions of people who hold certain formal and informal roles: characteristic patterns of conflict management, communication, and decision making between physicians and managers.

Open systems theory suggests that behaviors are influenced by structures, but also that structures are defined and redefined by the behavioral patterns of the people in them. Since behaviors are shaped by socialization into professions, for example, which occurs outside the organization's boundaries, we need all five levels of analysis to understand completely the full range of factors and processes, as well as their relative strengths, that influence physician and manager behaviors. Because individuals experience membership in many different social units *at the same time*, the open systems model helps us see that physicians and managers may be influenced in their interactions by *all* the levels, though the strength of each may vary as a result of both internal conditions and the local environment. Thus actions can be affected by the changes imposed by regulatory processes, purchaser actions, and societal demands on their profession; by their professional socialization; by the specific strategy and task structures of the organizations in which they work; by the specific relations among groups in their unit; and by the personalities and other characteristics of individual participants.

## Diagnosis Using the Open Systems Framework

The first step towards improving physician-manager relations in a specific organizational context is accurate and comprehensive diagnosis of the forces shaping the dynamics of that relationship. The discussion of the open systems model of organizations in this chapter suggests some general principles that can be applied in a systematic assessment of physician-manager relations in a health care setting:

- Any management problem in an organization is the result of multiple factors, so a solution based on a single theoretical perspective will be of limited utility because by definition it will overlook some of the forces at work. Physicians are certainly influenced by financial incentives, but they are influenced by other factors (such as professionalism) as well.

- Physician-manager tensions are caused by factors external to, as well as internal to, any particular organization.

- The specific pattern of physician-manager relations in any organization is part of a larger pattern of relationships among all the groups in that organization.

We could generate other such general open systems rules, but these are sufficient to illustrate our primary point: that managers hoping to improve physician-manager relations need to take an inclusive, multilevel approach to the problem. Starting from these principles, we can also develop some more specific guidelines about physician and manager roles in health care organizations.

- Physicians and managers *share* a concern that the organization serve the health care needs of its primary customers, patients. They are the focus of the physician's clinical responsibility, and serving them is his or her primary professional purpose. Managers must ensure that patients are satisfied with the responsiveness, cost, and quality of the care received because successful service is the principal source of the organization's viability. However, the manager's task is complicated by the fact that the organization also must serve at least two other customer groups: payers and the physicians themselves. Both are also interested in patient service but have other concerns as well. Payers want to limit their outlays; physicians want to concentrate on practicing good medicine.

• Some of the tensions between physicians and managers spring from the laudable desire of both to provide the best service to the customer, but *as measured by the norms of their own profession*. For example, physicians who interact directly with patients may give greater weight to responding to the patients' expressed desires for service than to cost. Managers, conversely, may emphasize the cost dimension more than physicians do. Thus a certain amount of conflict between physicians and managers in health care organizations must be expected and, if managed well, can be healthy. Their differing perspectives can serve the organization by helping it balance its obligations to all its customers.

• Although physicians and managers typically serve in separate hierarchical structures (Harris, 1977), the reality is that their worlds intersect continuously and at all levels. It cannot be otherwise in a complex human system, and if the organization is to provide excellent and reliable patient care then managers must be involved in the clinical arena, and physicians in administration. This interconnectedness must be deliberate and planned, however, not the result of idiosyncratic happenstance.

## Applying the Open Systems Approach to the Stories of Chapter One

To illustrate the diagnostic value of the open systems framework, we return to five of the stories of poor performance by health care organizations recounted in Chapter One. We use each of the five to illustrate in more detail one of the five open systems concepts reviewed earlier in this chapter. The framework helps us both to describe the nature of the breakdowns reflected in the stories and to understand more fully the stakes involved in each. As we will see in Chapter Nine, it can also help managers create remedies for those problems.

Not all of these stories concern relations between physicians and managers directly. However, the interdependence of physicians and managers in health care settings is apparent in all of them, and each points to the value of the open systems model as a diagnostic tool to improve organizational performance.

### Story One: Enrolling in an HMO

We use this story to discuss *boundary regulation*. Here, the boundary is the organizational boundary between would-be subscribers to the HMO and the HMO itself. In the story, a woman diagnosed with cancer attempted to obtain information from several HMOs about their coverage policies in order to choose one that would best suit her needs. It took this consumer a remarkably long time to reach the point of being able to make choices because she had so much trouble getting basic information about coverage.

At one level, this appears to be a straightforward story about sloppy boundary management resulting from organizational practices that have created an HMO boundary that is very difficult to permeate. Customers cannot easily get the information they need to make rational decisions about joining, and the difficult interactions with organizational representatives undoubtedly drive some frustrated consumers away.

But at another level, this story provides an example of how seemingly dysfunctional management systems (here, the obscurity of information about plan coverage) may serve some purpose for the organization. We do not have enough information to know for sure, but the HMOs in the story may simply be ignoring individual would-be subscribers in order to attend to more important corporate clients. Some might justify such a strategy by saying that the largest part of the business by far depends on service to groups, and therefore it is rational to focus on serving them well even if those who join as individuals get short shrift. Cynics would add that individual subscribers, like the woman who wrote the op-ed article, tend to be poorer medical risks and therefore "undesirable" customers, so complicating their inquiries—whether through inattention or by deliberately discouraging them—makes good business sense.

There is a downside to such a cumbersome intake system. For one thing, as portrayed in the newspaper article, it does not discriminate between good and bad risks. It appears that all callers have trouble getting information. Undoubtedly, some who are discouraged are good risks; some are probably members of groups who have a choice among several plans offered by their employer and are trying to clarify details about them before making a choice. In either event, the plan may be losing subscribers it would benefit from having.

We assume that the strategy of these organizations is to enroll as many customers as possible in order to maximize premium income, but to limit the money spent on their care. One could oversimplify it by saying it is based on volume (number of customers enrolled) and on profitability (controlling the cost of providing care to each member). This may be a defensible strategy so long as the organization is not deliberately discriminating against would-be subscribers on the basis of the expenses they are likely to require (the woman in the story would clearly be a high-cost subscriber).

Regardless, this strategy is a prescription for relationships of short duration. The practices signaled in the HMO intake process are bound to disappoint members and lose subscribers, including healthy ones. An HMO may be able to ignore an individual like the woman in our story with little long-term cost. However, it cannot afford to offend organizational purchasers offering many subscribers all of whom have choices among several plans. There is evidence that institutional as well as individual purchasers are becoming better informed and more demanding about the services provided to them.

This point brings us to the inherent interrelatedness between physicians and managers in this story, which on the surface appears to concern only administrative issues. This story can be read as a tale about *whose interests* determine the way the organizational boundary is regulated. It raises questions about how health care organizations have chosen to balance medical values (service to patient-customer) with financial values (service to payer-customer). It is possible, for example, that the screeners were deliberately trained to respond as they did (or at least that managers deliberately kept them in the dark about plan details). If that were the case, we may conclude that payers' short-term financial interests, rather than individual patient needs, shaped how the organizations screened potential customers. That is, intake processes may have been designed to keep costs down by discouraging high-cost individual shoppers, rather than by learning how to provide effective, cost-sensitive service to customers.

The marketing function bears directly on physician-manager relations, too. People who actually choose a plan in response to appealing representations from salespeople, whether over the phone or in face-to-face sessions at the workplace, do so because of expectations they form about the service they expect to obtain when they are sick. Instead of being withheld, sometimes information is distorted to present the most favorable picture possible of a plan's characteristics in order to attract, not discourage, subscribers. If doctors are unable to meet those expectations—if prior authorization procedures designed to discourage utilization are implemented—patients may become dissatisfied, not because the care is poor but because of the disconnection between the expectations fostered by salespeople trying to increase the numbers of subscribers and the care actually delivered by physicians.

## Story Two: Waiting to Be Seen

This is a story about *throughput*: a biker who had been hit by a car and was experiencing severe headaches waited for hours to be seen in his staff-model HMO. The story illustrates what can happen when patients present nonroutine demands for care to the administrative systems of health care organizations. Health care organizations "process" patients according to preestablished procedures, relying as much as possible on appointments scheduled in advance. That is the easiest way to bring the appropriate level and amount of resources to bear on a clinical problem without having either staff or facilities sitting idle. As in this case, however, it is not always possible to plan in advance, and a good health care organization must be able to respond appropriately to other requests for service. In many instances, when people "feel sick" and appear at the clinical office without an appointment, they can be "squeezed in" on a first come, first served basis. But as this story demonstrates, staff must be prepared to determine whether that approach is adequate in a particular instance, and when the patient's condition requires it, they must be able to respond.

This health care organization failed twice: first, it failed to provide competent urgent care to the biker by determining how serious his need was and whether his condition made it important for him to be seen promptly. In other words, they performed no triage function. He represented a nonroutine need for service. He did not call for an appointment, so staff could not arrange for him to come at a time convenient for them. Instead, he was dropped off by a good Samaritan. The organization's procedures should have included an initial determination about the seriousness of the patient's condition, especially given the possibility of a concussion.

Either no such system existed in this case or staff members (administrative, nursing, or medical) did not utilize it correctly. The doctor who would have treated the patient probably did not realize the biker was there, as he or she would be expecting only those patients who had scheduled appointments. In fact, physicians probably never set foot in the waiting room and therefore couldn't have seen the biker lying on the floor. Absent the physician's perspective on the nonroutine situation, the administrative systems were inadequate.

This story shows why both physicians and managers are essential in the process of designing and running systems to manage the clinical processes that form the core of the organization's operations. Physicians must set the standards for triaging and other basic procedures that assure appropriate patient care in routine *and nonroutine* circumstances alike.

The second failure occurred when the HMO staff failed to respond to obvious cues from the patient that he was having difficulty. He asked for aspirin for a severe headache, which should have triggered a series of questions about his condition. Later, he was so uncomfortable that he actually lay down on the floor because he could not hold his head up. Yet the HMO's staff did not respond. Ultimately, the biker experienced virtually no value from his HMO membership: this was not a solo practitioner's office, but it was his home practice. His own primary care physician, along with colleagues, practiced in that very space, and his medical record was readily available. Yet he might as well have been in a foreign country.

The organization must have procedures for treating unplanned patients appropriately, guided primarily by their medical condition—which must be determined first and foremost. Then staff must be monitored to determine that good care is being delivered according to the plans. Managers cannot establish adequate procedures alone. They need input from physicians in their role as clinical experts. What does a nonroutine patient treatment process need to accomplish, and what is the best way to organize it? This is another example of the value of a partnership between clinicians and managers.

**Story Three: "The Patient's Personal Physician"**

This is a story about *homeostasis* not yet achieved. Here, the physician deliberately left work without greeting and reassuring her young patient, who had arrived for care following a sports accident. This tale reveals two problems: first, the difficulties that can develop when complex and potentially conflicting professional role definitions are not clarified, and second, the need for management systems that ensure that an organization can learn from its mistakes. In the language of open systems, both are issues involving homeostasis because both illustrate the situation that develops in organizations *before* self-correcting mechanisms have been developed and are introduced.

As doctors are drawn to practice within health care organizations, especially when they become salaried employees, concerns have been expressed about their potential role confusion: will they start to behave like clock-watching functionaries instead of professionals whose commitment is to serve the health care needs of their patients, whatever the hour? This story shows that those who are concerned about this potential may have good reason to worry.

One of the defining characteristics of HMOs, especially the staff-model type, is that the patient picks a primary care physician who then takes responsibility for providing and/or managing care. In exchange for the benefit of having a personal physician with those obligations (and of having to pay only a fixed premium), the patient is granted access to the organization's services only through that physician. Thus the primary care physician serves two professional roles for the patient: the *personal physician*, who will uniformly assume clinical responsibility for her patients and with whom they ideally will form a close and trusting relationship; and the *gatekeeper*, who serves as an organizational agent in delivering basic health maintenance services and in monitoring patient access to health care services. In this case, the patient and her family expected a personal physician; the physician, in contrast, acted as if her gatekeeping role were primary and delegable to the covering physician on duty after five o'clock. Her income did not depend on maintaining the personal touch with her patient; nor would she be held accountable for her patient's dissatisfaction. Thus there was confusion about roles and expectations.

But the open systems framework suggests that the failure here is managerial as much as medical. True, the patient and her family were treated impersonally: the doctor acted as if her relationship with the patient were not important, and in so doing abrogated a fundamental principle of professional medical care. However, the organization did not help her, and by implication other physicians, by reinforcing her role as an autonomous professional as well as an organizational employee.

In this case, the teenager received the same first-level care—examination, pain relief, and a referral to an orthopedist—that she would have received in any case. The primary effect of the primary care physician's departure was to weaken the parents' ties to the HMO. Subsequently, the orthopedist's unresponsiveness to the patient's complaints prolonged the teenager's recovery period, and the family left the HMO.

It is a management responsibility to ensure that feedback is obtained routinely, and if in this case feedback about the family's dissatisfaction with either physician's behavior had reached the organization, we would have expected the managers to develop systems to keep this from happening again. However, neither physician had a personal stake in learning whether the patient and her family were happy with her treatment and so the physicians never knew of their complaints. In addition, the HMO, which at the time was still growing, was probably able to replace this family easily. Thus, there were few mechanisms in the system to allow the organization to learn from mistakes and to take corrective action. This story, and the subsequent departure of the patient's family, consequently represents a failure of management.

We said this was a story about homeostasis not yet achieved in health care organizations. The family's withdrawal may have been caused most directly by the behavior of the doctors, but it is the organization that bears the ultimate cost—at least if the story is repeated—and the organization is management's responsibility. If physicians need to learn new behaviors, or to conceptualize differently their professional roles in organizational settings, then managers must introduce systems to help them learn. We need to examine management processes that tolerate a primary care physician's avoiding her patient and leaving the building through a back door. Managers also must design routine actions—perhaps exit interviews for disenrolling subscribers—to capture information and feed it back into the organization, to prevent future mistakes.

## Story Four: Failing to Communicate

This is a story about confusion that occurs when *differentiation* in function is not clarified. A patient who was being treated for stomach distress called to ask a question about her treatment but never received a call in return. As a result, and on the advice of the clerk in a different unit who was responsible for scheduling the diagnostic procedure her physician had recommended, she decided not to undergo the procedure, which had been intended to rule out serious causes of the symptoms she was experiencing. Neither the physician nor anyone in her office ever inquired about whether she had undergone the procedure or whether her symptoms had subsided.

In this HMO, or at least on this unit, several categories of employee are responsible for returning patients' calls. In the absence of clear rules assigning call-backs to particular individuals, the system broke down. The breakdown reveals the vulnerability of patient care to lapses in administrative systems. Nor did the unit have a tickler file to alert clinical staff about whether expected events (here, a test that had been ordered) had in fact occurred.

The problem here could be understood as a failure to differentiate clinical tasks from administrative tasks. By one definition, returning this patient's call was a clinical task. It is the physician's responsibility to maintain a relationship with a patient, and the patient's questions were medical ones. By another definition, returning the call was an administrative task; having the nurse practitioner make the call is a less expensive use of resources, especially if she were able to respond to the patient's questions without involving the physician. If we assume the best, the failure occurred in a confusion between the physician and the nurse practitioner about who was supposed to return the call.

However, this story shows a potentially serious instance of confusion over differentiation in functions that, in retrospect, reveals that reliable management systems were absent from this unit. First, the patient should not have received advice about the diagnostic procedure from a nonclinical clerk answering the phone. This is a failure of management in not clearly defining the limits of the clerk's role and then monitoring performance. Second, there were no procedures to (1) determine who had responsibility to return this particular call, (2) be sure that *all* patient calls were returned, and (3) see that doctor-recommended courses of treatment were understood and followed. In the absence of simple role-definition and follow-up procedures, the patient felt she received inadequate attention.

In our discussion of open systems, we noted that one output was information about the organization's processes and activities, and that that information is used as feedback to make organization staff aware of adjustments that need to be made. In this case, although the patient had information about performance that could have been useful to conscientious managers, no one asked her for it, and she did not volunteer it. She was annoyed with her own too-frequent experience (apparently shared by many HMO customers) of having to take the role of the "information system" for physicians. That is, even though organizations create staff and management procedures to furnish patient information to physicians, clinicians often rely on patients to perform that function. The cardiac patient in Chapter Six had to perform that function several times over the course of an episode in which he saw several physicians, none of whom knew when he walked into the examining room why he had come—even though he had explained it to the scheduler and in one instance had been referred by another physician. Increasingly, good quality care requires that connections be made between several providers (sometimes in a single organization) or between patients and providers. The organization's managers—with the help of clinicians—must create differentiated roles and processes that assure that these tasks are accomplished.

## Story Five: Paying the Bill

We use this story to illustrate the need for *integration* across boundaries not only within health care organizations but also beyond the organization's walls. In the story, information authorizing the treatment of the patient was transferred appropriately to the payer, but apparently it was incomplete because authorization of use of an ambulance was not included. Neither the MCO nor the ambulance company recognized that comprehensive, cross-organizational communication about all aspects of the bill was an essential aspect of service to their customer. And no one was willing to exercise personal judgment to override the automated information system and make the assumption that since the physician had authorized use of the emergency room, she would have authorized use of transportation to get there.

This is still another example of problems that arise in customer service when clinical and administrative functions are not adequately integrated or coordinated. Here, administrative staff were trained to report authorized services to the payer. However, neither the clerks nor the supervisors to whom the patient complained were trained to exercise judgment about the organization's role in legitimizing to the insurance company *all* the patient's costs, including the ambulance ride. Both the ambulance company employee who did the paperwork and the MCO/insurer supervisor who was asked to respond failed to recognize that he or she was performing a key organizational role, as a kind of broker for patients, which had implications for the organization's reputation with its customers. And like the physician in "The Patient's Personal Physician," he or she probably had no idea that the patient would experience repeated frustration over the billing confusion, or that the patient would blame the HMO. Nor is it likely that the HMO employees understood—or considered it relevant to their work—that members might choose to leave the health plan over exactly this kind of frustration.

Since integration of clinical and administrative activities is a key element of good customer service, *all* health care professionals and other employees must be trained to think about issues beyond the narrow concerns of their own discipline or their own routine tasks. Everyone who works in the name of the organization—whether physicians, as in "The Patient's Personal Physician," or clerical staff, in this case—affects the organization's reputation with customers. If the interaction is unsatisfactory, repercussions will be felt. As the organization's custodians, managers are responsible for building a customer-focused organizational culture, training staff and others to treat everyone as a valued customer, and rewarding them when they do so.

## Conclusion

In this chapter, we have conceptualized health care organizations as open systems. Underlying this model is an assumption that everyone concerned with health care organizations—clinicians, managers, and consumers—must understand a problem thoroughly and accurately, in all its complexity, before they can solve it.

The test of whether the open systems framework, or any other model, is useful can be summarized with four pragmatic criteria:

1. *Validity:* the model must present an accurate (and therefore complex) view of environmental pressures, organizational structures, and individual tasks in health care organizations.

2. *Objectivity:* the model must hold both managers and physicians accountable for improving relations between them, without fixing blame exclusively on one group or the other.

3. *Realism:* the model must accurately reveal the fundamental goals and priorities of managers and physicians, both where they are congruent and where they diverge.

4. *Feasibility:* the framework must lead participants to ideas for improving organizational performance that are possible to implement given constraints on resources such as time, money, and professional attention.

The open systems framework satisfies these criteria. However, a useful model is only a tool that *permits* a proper diagnosis of the dimensions of the problem in each situation. The open systems model suggests that physician-manager relations are embedded in, and affected by, other managerial issues. Thus, we cannot attack the physician-manager question in isolation. Rather, we must look for solutions as part of a broader, systemic approach to a more complex set of challenges.

Finally, the most important practical step is to study and understand how effective health care managers, from the supervisory level to the CEO, are bringing this model to life so that good ideas can be transported to other organizations. Unfortunately, the health services research community has not yet provided much descriptive or explanatory research focused on the processes of care. Until more extensive research is available, we can offer only observations and our own analyses of cases with which we are familiar. Chapter Nine shows how some managers *are* working effectively with physicians and how some health care organizations have found ways to build collaborative physician-manager relations.

# 9

# The Problem-Solving Approach
## Creating Collaboration Between Physicians and Managers

In the preceding chapters we presented evidence from a wide range of sources showing a migration of health care consumers and physicians into organizational settings, a migration that is redefining the practice of medicine in the United States. Yet we also demonstrated that despite the sincere efforts of many, the performance of health care organizations is not meeting the expectations of these two major customer groups, patients and doctors. Finally, we argued that physician-manager collaboration is crucial to solving the performance problems evident in these organizations.

## Why Collaboration?

Why do we believe it is important that managers and physicians work together cooperatively? The first reason is that cost and quality assurance, which get so much attention in the general press, depend on it. Costs cannot be stabilized, nor quality assured, unless physicians and managers in health care organizations can work together. In part this is because the physician is now tightly coupled into the manager's universe. That is, the organization's success in meeting performance standards for quality, service, efficiency, effectiveness, and customer satisfaction depends largely on clinical decisions made by physicians. The stories in Chapters One and Six demonstrate clearly that a physician problem is an organizational problem.

Discussing the application of Total Quality Management (TQM) methods to health care organizations, Blumenthal and Edwards (1995) put it this way: "Many physicians have greeted the tenets of TQM with skepticism. . . . [Yet] because of physicians' central role in resource allocation decisions, . . . administrators of health care organizations will have to find ways to make their physicians active, committed supporters of TQM as an approach to improving organizational performance" (p. 229).

Second, the manager is also a key contributor to physician performance. In the stories we have recounted throughout this volume, including those we analyzed in more detail in Chapter Eight, what repeatedly looked at first like physician failure turned out to be managerial failure as well. In the complex world of ever more sophisticated treatments, which doctors are expected to deliver in ever shorter time for ever more constrained costs, the physician has to work smarter. But he or she also must depend on management for complete, accurate, and timely information; for creation and implementation of processes for the transfer of information between providers (doctor to doctor, doctor to pharmacy and back, doctor to hospital); for sufficient personnel and equipment, allocated effectively; and for appropriate administrative support. By providing those ingredients, managers make it possible for the processes of care to be smooth and seamless, as well as efficient and reliable.

Finally, health care organizations no longer have the luxury of taking time to work around the strains in physician-manager relations. The competitive and regulatory universe is changing too fast. Organizations that delay too long in making strategic and operational decisions jeopardize their own survival. Although managers must ensure that good decisions are made expeditiously, they *must* involve doctors in those decisions. The old patterns of physician-manager relations, which consisted primarily of conflict avoidance or political maneuvering, will not work any more.

# The Need to Involve Physicians

Doctors need to participate in organizational strategic decisions for two reasons. First, their primary expertise is in providing the services sought by the patients who are the health care organization's customers. Strategic decisions affect both who those patients are and what resources will be available to serve them. Second, if decisions are made without involving physicians, the message is clear: "You are not important. We made this decision without you, and we may make others as well. Just do as you are told!" This is not a message that inspires loyalty to the organization or encourages doctors to invest their energy or ideas. Nor is it paranoia if a physician worries about his or her expendability. When San Francisco Bay Area HMOs dropped hundreds of specialists from their rolls of authorized providers, they demonstrated dramatically to all physicians the reality of that worry (Russell, 1995). If managers think they can afford to ignore the sensibilities of physicians, let them try delivering services without doctors.

Despite evidence that the absence of effective cooperation between physicians and managers lies at the heart of many performance problems in health care organizations, little research—or even anecdotal evidence—is available to suggest that breakthroughs to improve physician-manager relations are on the horizon. On the contrary, as part of a large national study Shortell and his colleagues surveyed executives from thirty-three hundred hospitals recently and found that "only 14 percent of active staff physicians have been exposed to [TQM] training to date and only 10 percent have or currently are participating in a QI [quality improvement] project team" (Shortell et al., 1995, p. 207). Moreover, only a minority of hospitals (43 percent) "reported conducting at least some training in CQI/TQM" (p. 207), so physician involvement in these activities is really less than half of the 14 and 10 percent reported. Other findings indicated that "the vast majority of hospitals, over 70 percent, were not yet examining clinical processes or conditions to a significant extent" (Shortell et al., 1995, p. 208).

The situation may be somewhat better in MCOs, but it is obvious from the few available studies that major limitations obtain there as well. Gold, Hurley, Lake, Ensor, and Berenson (1995) conducted a telephone survey of CEOs and their designees in a sample of managed care plans (including several types of HMOs and PPOs) in each of twenty market areas throughout the country. Most reported using one or more methods of monitoring physician practice (clinically focused studies, physician profiling, utilization review, and practice guidelines) but also reported significant limitations in the data available to support these activities. While monitoring performance is a necessary component of quality assurance, it is not the same as engaging physicians in a collaborative process designed to develop and implement policies to ensure that good care is delivered reliably and efficiently. Finally, since only a small number of senior executives in each plan were interviewed, Gold and Hurley were not able to confirm what the plans' physicians actually experienced and what impact these activities had on their practice decisions.

A report by Blumenthal and Edwards (1995) on this last point is not encouraging. In six detailed case studies of leading integrated health systems, they found low involvement of physicians in TQM efforts. Confirming the point we made earlier, they write that "low involvement rates seemed to be related as much to management's reluctance to recruit physicians as to physicians' reluctance to participate though such physician resistance was present as well" (pp. 237–238). Kralewski (1995) reported recently on a detailed study of MCOs in the Twin Cities, which have consolidated into just a few organizations and which together have achieved a very high penetration in the local market. Echoing Shortell's finding about hospitals, Kralewski found that MCOs focus very little attention on the actual delivery of services, with only occasional feedback of information to physicians on their practice patterns. If that is the case in one of the most advanced managed care markets, it is unreasonable to expect more in markets that are less competitive.

### Causes of Physician-Manager Tensions

Do we understand why physicians and managers have found it difficult to collaborate? We think so, but there is little contemporary empirical research on physician-manager relationships to corroborate our views. Based on their survey of hospital executives, Shortell and colleagues (1995) identified a number of "barriers" to physician involvement in TQM activities: (1) doctors are skeptical about hospitals' motives; (2) many did not see the relevance of these approaches to their own practices; (3) they reported having too little time to participate; (4) relevant clinical data and analyses were lacking; (5) peer group support for physician involvement also was lacking; (6) some feared that formal quality improvement efforts, resulting in requirements for strict adherence to clinical protocols, might be used against them as malpractice threats (p. 217). If we are right about the need for physician-manager collaboration, then these obstacles to progress found by Shortell and colleagues mean that managers have much work to do: first, to persuade physicians that their primary motive is the same as physicians'—to serve patients well—and second, to begin the give-and-take process of actually negotiating with physicians to achieve an end state that both groups can support.

Although little relevant empirical work has been done in recent years on physician-manager relations, our review of the literature in Chapter Seven showed that useful conceptual explanations of physician-manager relations can be derived from five different theoretical perspectives. The bulk of the research conducted to date, however, has focused on macro-level issues, that is, on the formal, structural relations between groups of physicians and health care organizations (for example, Burns, Andersen, & Shortell, 1990; Gold, Hurley, Lake, Ensor, & Berenson, 1995). Although open systems theory offers a means of integrating organizational and intraorganizational perspectives on physician-manager relations with these more macro-level views, little has been written from this perspective.

### How to Improve Physician-Manager Collaboration

Can we see a way to improve relations? Yes. First, we can see glimpses of "best practices" in the literature. We know that some managers in some organizations are creating conditions in which physicians can practice more effectively and productively (see Blumenthal & Edwards, 1995, for example). However, more of these activities need to be documented, studied, evaluated, and reported, so that managers throughout the country can adapt them for local use. Second, the open systems model suggests a general diagnostic process that can help managers illuminate leverage points within their own organizations that they can exploit to produce change. These leverage points, which we explore in more detail in this chapter, offer some hope that physicians and managers might initiate projects that could change the pattern of their relations.

Finally, what will it take to get there? Since managers and physicians share responsibility for improving organizational performance and satisfying customers, they must make a commitment to work together, as trite as that may sound. However, it is the *role of managers* especially to foster an organizational climate of collaboration and to engage physicians in designing processes that can lead to that result. This means managers must study their own organizations—and their own behavior—to identify and implement initiatives to improve physician-manager relations. A major hurdle that managers must overcome is physicians' distrust of management, reinforced by managers' perceived focus on the bottom line and by their frequent choice to leave physicians out of key decisions.

## Points of Leverage in the Organization

What does it mean for managers to "create conditions" in which physician satisfaction and organizational performance will improve? What methods can they use toward that end? This question may seem easy enough to answer: everyone knows that managers can try to increase physician productivity via pay structures and employment contracts. However, treating the issue like a personnel problem that can be isolated and solved with an acceptable agreement about pay for hours worked is exactly the approach that has proved so unproductive to date. It represents an old-fashioned model of management that was discarded in most Fortune 500 companies a decade ago.

Corporate leaders in the most competitive companies know it takes more than simple monetary rewards to create among employees a sense of ownership in the organization's activities and accomplishments. Engaging employees in decisions that further the organization's mission is a management problem of the most complex form, embedded in all the other management and strategic challenges facing the organization. Yet researchers are finding that physicians are *not* being engaged by managers in these tasks (Blumenthal & Edwards, 1995; Shortell et al., 1995). One might ask, are physicians who practice in organizational settings being treated like the professional equivalent of assembly-line workers or mechanical deliverers of services, when employees on actual assembly lines are now being treated like key partners in producing organizational success? We believed they are, based on the discussion found in the previous chapters.

First, managers often start by assuming that physicians will not cooperate, leading them to prefer to manage at arms length, via formal reward and employment agreements. Why try to build a partnership with people who will only resist? (It is interesting that difficult labor relations problems seem to have been ameliorated only after managers were willing—or forced by competition or collective bargaining—to challenge their similar prejudices about blue collar workers.) From the physicians' side, a suspicion about the compromises on practice required in an organizational setting leads to a parallel arms-length attitude. Like academics, physicians expect to feel loyal to their profession rather than to an organization. Thus, the attitudes of managers and physicians reinforce each other, and in spite of their unhappiness, neither group is spontaneously moved to examine and challenge the historical hands-off patterns of interaction.

As Scott (1982) predicted, the natural tension between managerial and physician perspectives often leads to conflict. In many organizations, moreover, it seems that both parties would rather suffer than engage each other and manage these conflicts. Physicians, like other professionals, view nonclinical activity (particularly lengthy problem-solving meetings) as a waste of time. And managers are uncertain of their competence, if not their right, to comment on physician behavior. The distance between the two groups is preserved by the unwillingness of either to venture into the breech. As a result, physicians rarely have the opportunity to appreciate the sense of accomplishment that often follows a period of wrestling with organizational issues, and managers rarely experience the gratification that comes with success in facilitating cooperative problem solving.

The bad news, then, is that there are no easy, formulaic approaches to the challenge of creating a productive working relationship between physicians and managers in health care organizations. But the good news is that multiple avenues are available to work on the problem. We discuss several of these next.

### Strategy

Researchers and other observers are recognizing that, as institutional and individual customers demand more from health care organizations, involvement of physicians in the strategic planning process is more and more essential. For example, Wirth and Allcorn (1993) devote an entire chapter to joint hospital and medical group strategic planning efforts: "There is just too much complexity and too much at stake to not know what a hospital or medical group is trying to accomplish" (p. 49). All types of health care organizations can benefit from including the perspective of those individuals who have most contact with customers and on whose decisions organizational performance most depends.

Ultimately, the objectives of *any* strategic planning process are (1) better understanding of the customer and the competitive environment, (2) better analysis of the organization itself and its strengths and weaknesses, and (3) better utilization of information to improve the "fit" between the organization and its marketplace. Our analysis in Chapter Eight of the stories told in Chapter One shows that customers are often disappointed when the norms of the medical profession are not reflected in the operations of health care organizations (for example, in the stories "Enrolling in an HMO" and "The Patient's Personal Physician"). One payoff, therefore, for the organization whose managers actively involve practicing physicians (not just physician-managers) in strategic thinking is that managers come to understand more clearly what customers expect from a health care provider. Another benefit is that physicians may come to understand more fully the competitive forces that impact the organization, to appreciate the implications for its performance, and thus to support key initiatives (for example, TQM). A third benefit may be that managers and physicians may come to a shared understanding of the organization's priorities, an understanding that may promote more collaborative behaviors.

Involving a broader sample of physicians in strategic decision making requires investing resources in selecting, training, and covering for those who participate. Physician involvement, in groups or as individuals, in organizational strategy formulation can take several forms:

- In formal strategic planning processes, at senior and middle levels

- In quality assessment programs that focus on patient, employee, and physician satisfaction measures

- In sessions to review and recraft organizational mission statements

- In the collection and dissemination of information about innovative practices (both clinical and administrative) that can bring organizational operations into alignment with external forces and that can help physicians improve their service to patients

While some physicians decline to spend time on these efforts, others agree to participate if they believe that managers genuinely want to understand and integrate clinical thinking into strategy formulation. Managers whose actions create that belief increase physicians' sense of ownership of organizational processes and loyalty to the organization as a vehicle for achieving professional gratification, and in the process they unleash the physicians' energy and creativity in service of the organizational mission.

## Structure

Perhaps the most obvious leverage point for improving physician-manager relations is in organizational structure, the formal reporting and coordinating relationships of individuals and departments. As we and many observers have noted, health care organizations are like universities in maintaining dual hierarchical structures. In the most extreme cases, professionals report only to professionals and administrators report only to administrators up to the most senior levels, in which a chief of service may be the only physician sitting with other top managers in an executive group. This structure both creates and perpetuates the hands-off relations between professionals and managers lower in the organizational structure: professionals do not feel responsible to managers and managers do not feel authorized to attempt to influence professional behavior. Solutions to this dilemma have been described and proposed by several recent observers. One example is the program-focused management structure described by Charns and Tewksbury (1993). In a formal structure they call the Program Organization, all key personnel on a unit or service are accountable to the head of that program, rather than to "one of their own kind" in the separate professional hierarchies. This structure has been modified in some organizations to become a matrix, in which physicians, nurses, technicians, and administrators report both to a program head and also to a person trained in their own field. The advantages of such a structure are that professionals bring multiple perspectives into a collaborative process to jointly design, oversee, and evaluate the systems governing clinical processes on a unit. This approach encourages a more effective focus on customer service by integrating (in open systems terms) key professional services.

The disadvantages, according to the authors, may be territorialism in the organization by program (rather than by profession) and the resistance of some groups (nurses, for example) to report to other professionals (Charns & Tewksbury, 1993). Moreover, a structure may *permit* collaboration, but by itself it is rarely enough to produce it. Top leaders must insist—and often reinforce their insistence—that participants work together as the theorists intended.

Many health care organizations have worked to bridge the dual hierarchy using a variety of other mechanisms throughout the hierarchy. Some involve physicians at the highest governance levels, on boards. Some CEOs structure top management groups (including physicians) in a wide range of cross-functional initiatives. Charns and Tewksbury (1993) lay out a spectrum of integrative mechanisms that work at lower levels in the organization, of which the Program Organization is just one.

## Culture

As used in organizational settings, the term *culture* refers to very basic, often unspoken assumptions about who we are as an organization or as a group within the organization, what we are supposed to be doing, and why we do it (McCollom, 1993). Shared values reflect individuals' positive experience of working in that organization ("we do this work because it is rewarding and important") but also the negative feelings most employees experience, either as individuals or as functional groups, about work ("people in this job are always underappreciated").

The impact of an organizational culture that did not promote professional engagement by primary care physicians with individual patients was illustrated in "The Patient's Personal Physician," where the physician left the HMO's offices by the back door instead of stopping to check on her young patient waiting to be seen for an athletic injury. Reports of physician alienation in managed care settings are not uncommon, as we noted in Chapter Six. The lesson from the corporate world is clear: the more impersonally employees of any kind (physicians included) are treated, the more they will limit their *personal* investment in their job (Hackman & Oldham, 1980). The analogy to blue collar workers is strange yet informative: generally, employees who feel exploited will work only up to "the letter of the law." They will wait to be told what to do and will not take the initiative to solve even obvious problems. Employees who feel well-treated, by contrast, will define their role broadly and will extend themselves beyond the call of duty. In contemporary health care organizations, this point applies not only to employees, but also to physicians whose ties are through contracts. Certainly, subscribers to managed care organizations must be able to rely on their physicians' primary commitment to meet their medical needs as patients. Physicians who are alienated from their organizations cannot be depended upon to do so.

What does it take to motivate a key group of organizational service providers like physicians? The formalistic, arms-length management style referred to earlier is responsible for some of the alienation partly because it places demands for higher physician productivity above other goals. Rather than working collaboratively with physicians to find better ways to meet a variety of clinical and managerial challenges (such as smooth patient flow, timely information transfer, effective cost control, and reasonable physician work hours), managers often resort to trying to manipulate "levers" outside the clinical arena, for example, the number of patients doctors are expected to see every day.

Like other organizational groups, physicians need to be involved in designing their own jobs and crafting the conditions under which they will work. No group can be expected to take more than perfunctory responsibility for organizational outcomes if they are not invited to participate in decisions that impact their work. This is especially true of professionals who have a long-standing tradition of attending only to professional work. Physicians are not experienced organizational members and have not learned the payoffs of involvement in decision making. Faced with unreasonable management practices, they are likely to withdraw even further into their clinical work. And the more managers perpetuate the division of decision making between clinical and managerial turf, the stronger the culture of alienation will become.

Managers and physicians need to make the effort to change the patterns of relations between their groups. Managers must take the lead in proposing sensible processes to involve physicians in problem solving; leaders throughout the organization, beginning at the top, must also convey through their actions an attitude that demonstrates their understanding that they depend on physicians to produce the organization's primary product, its medical services. As corny as it sounds, insisting on mutual respect (in behaviors as well as policies) is the first step to building a culture of customer responsiveness. This respect begins with an understanding of the legitimate differences between physicians' and managers' perspectives. A manager may have one perspective on how many patients a physician should see per day; physicians may have a different view. Until these different perspectives can be understood and accepted as legitimate for that group, rather than treated as evidence of ignorance, laziness, or manipulation, relations will not improve. This mutual appreciation can only come with face-to-face contact and discussion; it will never materialize in a hands-off culture.

## Management Systems

Management systems are the mechanisms and procedures used to coordinate across organizational units and functions. They include information systems, financial control systems, human resource policies, and administrative systems of all types. They involve scheduling procedures, materials control policies, patient intake criteria, and billing processes. In open systems terms, they are important means for achieving integration and efficiency. The more complex the organization, the more sophisticated its systems must be to produce reliable, high-quality outcomes.

The stories discussed in Chapter Eight show that management systems can be a powerful tool to improve physician-manager coordination, thereby improving organizational performance. An example from the previous chapter was the integrated and physician-accepted information system: integrated in that the same system links patient records, billing, and diagnostic results, and physician-accepted in that the system is actually utilized by clinicians. Managers trying to implement those systems have discovered not just that it is difficult and expensive to build them, but also that it is difficult to get physicians to use them.

To participate in the design and implementation of these systems, physicians need training and assistance in developing their own office management techniques to produce relatively fail-safe patient care arrangements. It is the role of managers to take the lead in purchasing and implementing these systems and to engage physicians at all stages of the process, beginning with articulation of the goals to be achieved.

## Staff

Staffing, like other functions in health care organizations, is complex. Employees range from part-time, low-skilled hourly workers to blue collar, pink collar and white collar technicians and lab, kitchen, and office workers to clinical professionals such as nurses and social workers to highly paid physicians and executives. Everyone who works in the name of the organization—whether physicians, as in "The Patient's Personal Physician" or the clerical staff in "Paying the Bill"—affects the organization's reputation with customers. If the interaction is unsatisfactory, repercussions will be felt. As the organization's custodians, managers are responsible for building a customer-focused organizational culture, training staff and others to treat everyone as a valued customer, and rewarding them when they do so.

These stories, along with others, illustrate the problems created in organizations in which individuals with a wide variety of educational backgrounds must work together. Health care professionals—nurses, technicians, physicians, managers—are trained intensively in a well-defined set of professional skills and perform their jobs using a predictable set of perspectives. Since integration of clinical and administrative activities is a key to customer service, *all* health care professionals and other employees must be trained to think beyond the boundaries of their own discipline.

The recruitment of physicians into key executive roles in organizations is evidence that boundary spanning across professional roles is recognized as a crucial function. This trend may be aided by curriculum changes in medical schools to include courses in health care economics and finance and managed care administration. In addition, physicians in midcareer are returning to school in increasing numbers for management degrees. Important as it can be to have managers who have practiced medicine, however, their clinical colleagues tend to view physician-managers more as managers than as physicians who bring the perspective of the practitioner into deliberations designed to result in organizational decisions (Heineke & Davidson, 1993). Moreover, our stories illustrate that training about legitimate organizational practices and interests must be offered to other groups within health care organizations.

In "Waiting to Be Seen," the nonclinician behind the reception desk needed to recognize the patient's need for prompt attention and exert herself to see that his clinical needs were met first, by bringing them to the attention of those who could provide the care he needed promptly.

## Implementation and the Open Systems Model

The leverage points discussed so far in this chapter are generalized, perhaps frustratingly so for managers looking for concrete suggestions. But the open systems framework tells us that specific recommendations need to be different for each organization and each situation. Formulas will not work. What we *can* do is point managers toward some productive arenas for change, ask them to think in systems terms, and encourage them to launch initiatives that test these ideas. Specific change efforts, however, must be built on careful analysis and diagnosis of conditions *in their own organization*. To assist managers in making some of the changes we suggest here, we present a *three-step process* for making change.

### Step One: Organizational Assessment

In order to develop an action plan, managers must look *into* their organization in some detail and ask a series of questions both about management climate (the soft side) and also about operations (the hard side):

•   On the soft side: What is the current state of relations between physicians and managers? What assumptions do these groups seem to hold about each other? For example, do managers tend to assume that physicians are uncooperative? Do physicians tend to assume that managers' motivation is always to squeeze more from them? What is the history of the relationship between the groups? Is the managerial culture participatory? Autocratic? What message do leaders send through their behaviors and words about what is important in the organization? Is the climate respectful? How is conflict typically managed?

- On the hard side: What are the responsibilities of the medical hierarchy? What responsibilities are lodged in the management structure? At what points in the organization do physician and management structures intersect? How well do these bridging structures work? Where are management systems helpful to clinical practice and where do they break down? How well is the organization measuring performance and on what variables? What strategy is the organization pursuing and how well does it fit with customer service objectives?

At this point, the connections between the soft and hard sides of the organization should become apparent. Once a manager can see the ways in which human relations issues connect to financial, information, and operational systems in the organization, she or he can begin to predict the impact of new initiatives on physician-manager relations.

### Step Two: Picking a Place to Start

At a more concrete level, managers then need to choose an arena for new initiatives. One approach is to compare a particularly problematic unit with a unit that seems to be working well. Starting with the latter, it is useful to assess the current "balance of power" on that unit: what aspects of the organization's work do physicians control? How do managers exercise influence? Specific operational issues range from patient intake to physician work load, facility staffing and hours, and the use of diagnostic routines to quality assessment processes. Diagnostic questions might include:

- On this unit, how does management currently support physician practice?

- How effective is this influence in facilitating good clinical operations and customer satisfaction?

- How effective is this support in producing physician satisfaction?

- In what ways are physicians involved in management decisions?

- What objectives do the groups seem to share? On what objectives do they seem to differ?

This assessment should provide a picture of how a balance can be struck between good clinical operations and physician satisfaction. To sharpen the image, it is useful to pick a problematic unit (measured by utilization rates, high turnover of patients or staff, or another concrete indicator) and conduct the same type of assessment.

### Step Three: Choosing a Direction for Change

Generally, there are two strategies for managers acting as change agents in complex systems, one involving higher risk than the other. The high-risk strategy is to pick a problematic area as a pilot, invest in a comprehensive assessment and change effort, and demonstrate both a collaborative approach and dramatic improvement (by objective measures). If the project is successful, the message quickly spreads to the rest of the organization that management intervention can improve clinical operations. The risk lies in the *if*. The effort can fail if the problem is very difficult, if the managers or physicians are not good "process" people, or if sufficient resources are not made available.

A lower-risk strategy is to launch several lower-profile initiatives in a variety of locations in the organization. This approach allows managers to test several types of interventions—new team structures, cross-training, flexible physician workloads—to see which are most effective and which might be most easily disseminated more widely throughout the organization.

In either scenario, managers must understand and follow basic rules for leading change in complex systems (Beckhard and Harris, 1987; Mohrman et al., 1989). Guidelines that seem particularly relevant here are:

- Put together a multidisciplinary group to lead the effort. Signal in the composition of the group that both physicians and managers will be represented by members respected by their peers. Set the tone in the leadership group for collaborative relations.

- State the objectives of the change initiative clearly and let the affected parties comment. Be willing to modify them. Don't overpromise.

- Share information: Make the results of an initial assessment available to unit members, listen to them, and respond to their reactions. Know that people will be more likely to support change if they can provide input.

- Don't work uphill. Pick projects that are likely to succeed and use leaders who are respected. Charge the group members with working it through. Provide the leaders with training in group problem solving. At the same time, choose *real* problems to work on. Don't waste people's time.

- Set a timetable: if you have to renegotiate it, do it publicly.

## Real Cases: Two Examples of Change Efforts

To make the point that change *is* possible and that physicians and managers *can* find good results in collaborative efforts, we present two examples reported by Blumenthal and Edwards (1995) in which multidisciplinary teams produced new and better ways of delivering care. In one case, the initiative came from a doctor; in the other, it came from managers. In both, managers created conditions in which group attention to clinical problems, including the use of resources in delivering care, was encouraged and facilitated.

❖ ❖ ❖ ❖ ❖ ❖ ❖

## The Hip and Knee Replacement Team at Henry Ford

"The hip and knee replacement team at Henry Ford Hospital began as one surgeon's desire to match what he saw as best practice at another hospital. He convened a group of physicians, nurses, social workers, discharge planners, and health plan administrators who were involved in the care of joint-replacement patients to look at ways to improve the processes of care. The team had the dual goals to improve care by standardizing methods and to improve satisfaction of those people working with joint-replacement patients. Lacking any formal TQM training, the groups took about four months to begin to work together effectively as a team. However, within one year, they had redesigned the care process and had begun treating one surgeon's patients under the new protocol. After a few months of tracking these patients, all three surgeons adopted the same care plan. The revised approach emphasized standardizing preoperative tests and increasing patient education about their expected recovery program. Postoperative care by trained nurses was increased as well.

"After the intervention, inpatient days decreased from a range of seven to ten days per stay to five days. Once home, patients worked with home health nurses to chart their mobility progress and faxed this information to the surgeon. As a result of the intervention, joint-replacement patients were more satisfied with their care. At the time of the study, no adverse outcomes had been documented, and problems were being recognized on a more timely basis.

"The team was in the process of assessing the financial impact of shifting patients from inpatient to home care. Some participants in this team were now beginning to investigate ways to improve the functioning of the operating room" (Blumenthal & Edwards, 1995, pp. 244–245. Reprinted with permission.).

❖ ❖ ❖ ❖ ❖ ❖ ❖

## Planning to Improve Care of Pediatric Asthma at Harvard Community Health Plan (HCHP)

"As part of a strategic plan to improve quality of care, managers of HCHP assembled a pediatric advisory group to examine pediatric care in the Health Centers Division, the division responsible for its staff-model HMO. The pediatric team identified asthma care as an area needing attention because of the high rates of emergency room visits and hospitalization among asthma patients. An asthma team was formed that identified a particular goal: to redesign the medical records of pediatric asthmatics to support chronic and acute asthma management in a way consistent with newly released national asthma guidelines. Using the revised record, all pediatricians would be prompted to reduce variation in management in all settings, encourage inter-provider communication, coordinate patient and family education with other aspects of asthma management, and provide clinicians the opportunity to monitor the patients' functional status in a standardized way.

"The team members included five pediatricians, an allergist, three physician managers, a director of information services, an analyst, and a nonclinical facilitator. They began by breaking the original project into manageable subproblems. The team followed a formal TQM approach: identifying problems with the current system, brainstorming solutions, defining and surveying its customers, and identifying process improvements.

"The team began its work in January 1992 and met regularly until the time when they proposed changes to the electronic medical record (about nine months). As a result, they won the Schering Laboratories Tribute to Excellence Award for their work in developing a process to improve asthma care. They had expected to begin piloting the new medical record system by the summer of 1993, but at the time of the study the necessary changes in the computerized medical record had not been implemented, so there were no results to report. Meanwhile, the group had moved on to address other asthma concerns, including guideline distribution, baseline measurement, and the design of clinician and patient education programs" (Blumenthal & Edwards, 1995, pp. 246–247. Reprinted with permission.).

♦ ♦ ♦ ♦ ♦ ♦ ♦

These cases can teach us some practical lessons:

- The initiative to solve problems can come from physicians or managers. If physicians take the initiative, managers must be prepared to respond with tangible encouragement.

- Group efforts take time. The problems often need to be subdivided and redefined, data need to be assembled and analyzed, and potential solutions need to be ironed out through the give-and-take process in the group. It also takes time because at first the participants are a group in name only, and they will need to overcome natural suspicions, misunderstandings, and normal resistance to change in order to transform themselves into a team.

- Clear, focused goals are important. Also, the initial goals may get transformed into more useful ones as the group proceeds.

- Group leadership is needed, either in the form of a designated facilitator or a leader within the group whose primary focus is on defining and solving the problem.

- Resources are required: time, money, and, very importantly, relevant information.

- Senior management must support the process, because meeting over an extended period is expensive and implementation of the agreed-upon solution may require an additional investment.

- Progress for the organization as a whole is made one step at a time—problem by problem, group by group.

## Conclusions

Throughout this book we have talked about physicians and managers in rather global terms. In this chapter, we showed that physician-manager collaboration develops through actions taken to solve specific problems, step by step. Physicians are essential participants in these initiatives. They are not unfamiliar with diagnosis and implementation as processes. They use them all the time in the clinical arena.

Moreover, as Blumenthal and Edwards (1995) point out, physicians are comfortable with the scientific method, which involves testing hypotheses on the basis of information. Thus, while physicians' professionalism is often identified as an obstacle to collaboration with managers in problem-solving teams, it may also have advantages that can be exploited by skilled managers. The adoption and implementation of TQM or CQI processes may be a particularly fitting approach, as Blumenthal suggests. In the process, physician ties to the organization can be strengthened as they become engaged in efforts to improve the organization's ability both to serve its customers (their patients) and to survive in an increasingly hostile, competitive health care world.

Since physicians' primary professional commitment is and must be to serving their patients, managers can engage them in the organization's work by communicating their concern that the organization (not the individual physician, but the organization as a whole) is not serving its patients as well as possible or that their ability to continue to serve them well depends on making adjustments in patterns of caregiving. Managers focus problem-solving efforts on particular clinical problems, which are often at the core of organizational problems—a hospital that spends more money to treat hip-replacement patients than Medicare pays, or an HMO that has too many patients using expensive urgent care services after normal working hours. Managers who do engage physicians in problem-solving efforts must be willing to invest the resources needed to define the problem fully and then to solve it, even if the solution requires an additional investment.

Writing about HMOs, one author made the point that "HMOs must be developed and managed with the long-term goal of building a successful health care business, rather than short-term objectives of securing market share, income to providers, or financial write-offs" (Katz, 1993, p. 262). Accumulation of successes like those reported in the two brief cases above defines an organization that delivers good care reliably and efficiently in response to the needs of patients. The only way these successes can be achieved is if managers and physicians break down the barriers that keep them from working together effectively.

We have seen throughout this book that theory *can* be a helpful guide to managerial action. The open systems framework gives us insight into the specific dynamics of particular organizations and provides the basis for assessment and change. In this chapter, we have pointed to some of the arenas in which managers can act to create more collaborative relations with physicians. The purpose of these interventions is to improve clinical operations, organizational performance, and, not incidentally, physician satisfaction.

We have argued that many managers in health care organizations have been using approaches to problem solving that are too narrow for the complexity of the contemporary American health care system. Leaving physicians alone in their clinical arena, although that may be what both groups say they would prefer, will not produce either reliable health care or good organizational outcomes on other dimensions. Managers *must* engage physicians in multiple organizational arenas, for the good of patients, physicians, and the organization itself.

For their part, physicians must learn how to work *inside* organizations. In particular, they must understand that time invested in management efforts will pay off in improved practice conditions. The alienated-worker stance in organizations is self-perpetuating, and no one benefits from it. The more physicians become involved in organizational issues outside the care of their own patients, the more their personal and professional values will influence the organization.

No one said it would be easy, but if nothing else, it should be clear now that it is both essential and possible for managers and doctors to collaborate for the benefit of their patients, their organizations, the health care system, and themselves. Only if they do so will we have healthy health care organizations that can succeed in meeting the health care needs of Americans at the turn of the twenty-first century.

# Notes

## Chapter Two

1. The drop was 693, or 11 percent, from the high point of 6,310 in 1975.

2. The number of nonfederal community hospital beds declined from 4.2 per 1,000 population in 1972 to 3.6 per 1,000 in 1992.

## Chapter Three

1. It is worth noting there is evidence that primary care physicians value the relationship with patients, too. Freidson discusses this element (1970, p. 103), and Heineke and Davidson (1993) found it in their study of primary care physicians in a staff-model HMO.

2. The difference in total cost was $38.53 per month ($537.94 minus $499.41); but the difference in the employee's share was $85.49 ($255.29 minus $169.80).

## Chapter Four

1. This issue has an ethical dimension as well, which is beyond the scope of this work. See Jonsen, 1990; Gray, 1991; Rodwin, 1993.

2. Some argue that doctors can create their own demand and, at least in a fee-for-service system, reduce the loss that would result from the increase in the physician/population ratio. Part of the argument is that physicians have a target income and will increase work and

fees in order to earn that income. See, for example, Feldstein, 1970;
Evans, 1973; and Wilensky and Rossiter, 1983.

## Chapter Five

1. See Jonsen (1990), *The New Medicine and the Old Ethics*, in which
   he discusses how medical ethics must be updated to take account
   of conditions that did not apply when Hippocrates promulgated
   his oath.

2. Madison and Konrad (1988) also proposed a model of organizational
   structure within large group practices. They categorized group practices using similar terms: individualistic autonomous, administered
   autonomous, and heteronomous structures.

## Chapter Six

1. Staff-model HMOs used salary/bonus arrangements; group- and network-model HMOs often used special-purpose funds and withholding, calculating deficits and surpluses for the group as a whole; and
   IPA-model HMOs were split between fee-for-service and capitation
   systems, with withholdings and bonuses that varied considerably.

2. Nonetheless, the use of financial incentives raises ethical concerns
   too, since a physician's financial interest could be in conflict with
   the duty to care for the patient. While these issues are beyond the
   scope of our work, research on financial incentives must take note
   of them (Gray, 1991; Rodwin, 1993).

# References

Abbott, A. (1988). *The system of professions: An essay on the division of expert labor.* Chicago and London: The University of Chicago Press.

Abel-Smith, B. (1988). The rise and decline of the early HMOs: Some international experiences. *The Milbank Quarterly, 66*(4), 694–719.

Abrahamson, M. (1964). The integration of industrial scientists. *Administrative Sciences Quarterly, 9*(2), 208–218.

Alexander, J. A., & Morrisey, M. A. (1988). Hospital-physician integration and hospital costs. *Inquiry, 25,* 388–401.

Alper, P. R. (1987). Medical practice in the competitive market. *The New England Journal of Medicine, 316*(6), 337–339.

Alper, P. R. (1994). Primary care in transition. *Journal of the American Medical Association, 272*(19), 1523–1524.

Alt-White, A., Charns, M., & Strayer, R. (1983). Personal, organizational and managerial factors related to nurse-physician collaboration. *Nursing Administration Quarterly, 8*(1), 8–18.

Altman L. K., with E. Rosenthal. (1990, February 18). Changes in medicine bring pain to healing profession. *The New York Times,* p. 1.

Anders, G. (1990, June 20). Split Diagnosis. *The Wall Street Journal,* p. A1.

Asinof, L. (1990, June 21). [Untitled.] *The Wall Street Journal*, p. A1.

Baker, L. C., & Cantor, J. C. (1993). Physician satisfaction under managed care. *Health Affairs*, Supplement, 258–270.

Baker, L. C., Cantor, J., Miles, E., & Sandy, L. (1994, June). What makes young HMO physicians satisfied? *HMO Practice*, pp. 53–57.

Becker, E. A. (1994, December 25). Doctors bear all risks. *The New York Times*, News of the Week Section, p. 8.

Beckhard, R., & Harris, R. (1987). *Organizational transitions*. Reading, MA: Addison-Wesley.

Begun, J. W. (1985, Spring). Managing with professionals in a changing health care environment. *Medical Care Review, 42*(1), 3–10.

Begun, J. W., Luke, R. D., & Pointer, D. D. (1990). Structure and strategy in hospital-physician relationships. In S. S. Mick & Associates (Ed.), *Innovations in health care delivery: Insights for organization theory* (pp. 116–143). San Francisco: Jossey-Bass.

Benson, K. (1973, Summer). The analysis of bureaucratic-professional conflict: Functional versus dialectical approaches. *The Sociological Quarterly*, pp. 376–394.

Berenson, R. A. (1991). A physician's view of managed care. *Health Affairs, 10*(4), 106–119.

Berwick, D. M. (1988). Measuring and maintaining quality in a health maintenance organization. In K. Lohr and R. Rettig (Eds.), *Quality of Care and Technology Assessment*. Washington, DC: NAS Press.

Berwick, D. M., & Coltin, K. (1986). Feedback reduces test use in a health maintenance organization. *Journal of the American Medical Association, 255*(11), 1450–1454.

Betson, C., & Pedroja, A. T. (1989). Physician managers: A description of their jobs in hospitals. *Hospital and Health Services Administration, 34*(3), 353–369.

Bettner, M., & Collins, F. (1987). Physicians and administrators: Inducing collaboration. *Hospital and Health Services Administration, 32*(2), 151–160.

Blendon, R. J., Benson, J. M., et al. (1993). *A survey of American attitudes toward health care reform*. Princeton, NJ: Robert Wood Johnson Foundation.

Blumenthal, D., & Edwards, J. (1995). Involving physicians in total quality management: Results of a study. In D. Blumenthal & A. C. Scheck (Eds.), *Improving clinical practice: Total quality management and the physician* (pp. 229–266). San Francisco: Jossey-Bass.

Blumenthal, D., & Scheck, A. C. (Eds.) (1995). *Improving clinical practice: Total quality management and the physician*. San Francisco: Jossey-Bass.

Bock, R. (1988). Sounding board: The pressure to keep prices high at a walk-in clinic: A personal experience. *New England Journal of Medicine, 319*(12), 785–787.

Bowen, D. (1982). Toward a viable concept of assertiveness. In D. T. Hall, D. Bowen, R. Lewicki, and F. Hall (Eds.), *Experiences in management and organizational behavior*, (3rd ed., pp. 332–335). New York: Wiley.

Bowman, M., & Gross, M. L. (1986, September–October). Overview of research on women in medicine: Issues for public policymakers. *Public Health Reports*, pp. 513–521.

Boyatzis, R. E., Cowen, S. S., Kolb, D. A., & Associates. (1994). *Innovation in professional education: Steps in a journey from teaching to learning*. San Francisco: Jossey-Bass.

Brailer, D. J., & Van Horn, R. L. (1993). Health and the welfare of U.S. business. *Harvard Business Review, 71*(2), 125–132.

Burns, L. R., Andersen, R. M., & Shortell, S. M. (1989). The impact of corporate structures on physician inclusion and participation. *Medical Care, 27*(10), 967–982.

Burns, L. R., Andersen, R. M., & Shortell, S. M. (1990). The effect of hospital control strategies on physician satisfaction and physician-hospital conflict. *Health Services Research, 25*(3), 527–560.

Carton, B. (1995, January 6). What's up, Doc? Stress and counseling. *The Wall Street Journal*, p. B1.

Cashman, S., Parks, C., Ash, A., Hemenway, D., & Bicknell, W. (1990). Physician satisfaction in a major chain of investor-owned walk-in centers. *Health Care Management Review, 15*(3), 47–57.

Charns, M. P., & Schaefer, M. J. (1983). *Health care organizations: A model for management.* Englewood Cliffs, NJ: Prentice-Hall.

Charns, M. P., & Tewksbury, L. S. (1993). *Collaborative management in health care: Implementing the integrative organization.* San Francisco: Jossey-Bass.

Cherner, L. L. (1993). *The universal healthcare almanac.* Phoenix: Silver & Cherner.

Chuck, J. M., Nesbitt, T. S., Kwan, J., & Kam, S. M. (1993). Is being a doctor still fun? *Western Journal of Medicine, 159*(6), 665–669.

Cimini, M. H., & Behrmann, S. L. (1992). Collective bargaining, 1991: Recession colors talks. *Monthly Labor Review, 115*(1), 21–33.

Coburn, D. (1992). Freidson then and now: An "internalist" critique of Freidson's past and present views of the medical profession. *International Journal of Health Services, 22*(3), 497–512.

Congressional Budget Office. (1991). *Rising health care costs: Causes, implications and strategies.* Washington, DC: U.S. Government Printing Office.

Cummings, T., & Huse, E. (1989). *Organizational development and change.* 4th ed. New York: West.

Davidson, S. M. (1982). Physician participation in Medicaid: Background and issues. *Journal of Health Politics, Policy and Law, 6*(4), 703–717.

Davidson, S. M. (1992, April). Competition and health care reform. Working Paper 92–48, Boston University School of Management.

Delbecq, A., & Gill, S. (1985). Justice as a prelude to teamwork in medical centers. *Health Care Management Review, 11*(4), 45–51.

Deming, W. E. (1986). *Out of the crisis.* Cambridge, MA: MIT Center for Advanced Engineering Study.

Derzon, R. A. (1988). The odd couple in distress: Hospitals and physicians face the 1990s. *Frontiers of Health Services Management, 4*(3), 4–19.

Deutsch, M. (1973). *The resolution of conflict*. New Haven, CT: Yale University Press.

Eckholm, E. (1994, December 18). While Congress remains silent, health care transforms itself. *The New York Times*, pp. 1, 34.

Eisenberg, J. M. (1986). *Doctors' decisions and the cost of medical care*. Ann Arbor, MI: Health Administration Press.

Ellwood, P. M., Enthoven, A. C., & Etheredge, L. (1992). The Jackson Hole initiatives for a twenty-first century American health care system. *Health Economics, 1*, 149–169.

Emery, R. E., & Trist, E. L. (1965). The causal texture of organizational environments. *Human Relations, 18*, 21–32.

Enthoven, A. (1993). The history and principles of managed competition. *Health Affairs*, Supplement, 24–48.

Enthoven, A., & Kronick, R. (1989). A consumer-choice health plan for the 1990s: Universal health insurance in a system designed to promote quality and economy. *The New England Journal of Medicine, 320*(1), 29–37; 320(2), 94–101.

Evans, R. G. (1973). Supplier-induced demand: Some empirical evidence and implications. In M. Perlman (Ed.), *The economics of health and medical care* (pp. 162–173). London: MacMillan.

Feldstein, M. S. (1970). The rising price of physicians' services. *The Review of Economics and Statistics*, 121–133.

Flood, A. B., Scott, W. R., Ewy, W., & Forrest, W. H., Jr. (1982). Effectiveness in professional organizations: The impact of surgeons and surgical staff organizations on the quality of care in hospitals. *Health Services Research, 17*(4), 341–377.

Foulkes, F. (1987). The Honeywell case. Boston University School of Management.

Fox, P. D., Heinen, L., & Steele, R. J. (1986). *Determinants of HMO success*. Washington, DC: Office of Health Maintenance Organizations, U.S. Public Health Service.

Freidson, E. (1970). *Profession of medicine*. Chicago: University of Chicago Press.

Freidson, E. (1973). Prepaid group practice and the new demanding patient. *Milbank Quarterly, 51*(4), 473–488.

Freidson, E. (1985). The reorganization of the medical profession. *Medical Care Review, 42*(1), 11–35.

Frese, M. (1982). Occupational socialization and psychological development: An underemphasized research perspective in industrial psychology. *Journal of Occupational Psychology, 55*, 209–224.

Freudenheim, M. (1995, July 2). States shelving ambitious plans on health care: More people uninsured. *The New York Times*, pp. 1, 20.

Fried, B. (1989). Power acquisition in a health care setting: An application of strategic contingencies theory. *Human Relations, 41*(12), 915–927.

Gabel, J., DiCarlo, S., Sullivan, C., & Rice, T. (1990). Employer-sponsored health insurance, 1989. *Health Affairs, 9*(3), 161–175.

Gabel, J., Liston, D., Jensen, G., & Marsteller, J. (1994). The health insurance picture in 1993: Some rare good news. *Health Affairs, 13*(1), 327–336.

Gilbert, S. M. (1995). *Wrongful death: A medical tragedy.* New York: Norton.

Glandon, G. L., & Morrisey, M. A. (1986). Redefining the hospital-physician relationship under prospective payment. *Inquiry, 23*, 166–175.

Gold, M., Hurley, R., Lake, T., Ensor, T., & Berenson, R. (1995). *Arrangements between managed care plans and physicians: Results from a 1994 survey of managed care plans.* Washington, DC: Physician Payment Review Commission.

Goldman, L. (1990). Changing physicians' behavior: The pot and the kettle. *The New England Journal of Medicine, 322*(21), 1524–1525.

Goss, J. (1961). Influence and authority among physicians in an outpatient clinic. *American Sociological Review, 26*, 39–51.

Goyert, G. L., Bottoms, S. F., Treadwell, M. C., & Nehra, P. C. (1989). The physician factor in cesarean birth rates. *The New England Journal of Medicine, 320*(11), 706–709.

Grafe, W. R., McSherry, O. R., Finkel, M. L., & McCarthy, E. G. (1978). The elective surgery second opinion program. *Annals of Surgery, 188*(3), 323–330.

Gray, B. H. (1991). *The profit motive and patient care.* Cambridge, MA: Harvard University Press.

Griffith, J. R. (1993). *The moral challenges of health care management.* Ann Arbor, MI: Health Administration Press.

Grimm, R. H., Shimoni, K., Harlan, W. R., & Estes, E. H. (1975). Evaluation of patient-care protocol use by various providers. *The New England Journal of Medicine, 292*(10), 507–511.

Grossman, G. M. (1992). U.S. workers receive a wide range of employee benefits. *Monthly Labor Review,* pp. 6–43.

Hackman, R., & Oldham, G. (1980). *Work redesign.* Reading, MA: Addison-Wesley.

Harris, J. F. (1977). The internal organization of hospitals: Some economic implications. *Bell Journal of Economics, 8*(2), 467–482.

Health Insurance Association of America. (1992). *Sourcebook.* Washington, DC: Health Insurance Association of America.

Heineke, J. (1992). *The effect of operations strategic decisions on obstetric processes and outcomes in health maintenance organizations.* Doctoral dissertation, Boston University School of Management.

Heineke, J., & Davidson, S. M. (1993). Physician-manager relationships: An empirical investigation. Proceedings of the Northeast Decision Sciences Institute, Philadelphia, March 31–April 2, 1993, pp. 225–227.

Heineke, J., & Meile, L. C. (1989). Managing in the health care industry. Unpublished working paper, Babson College.

Hemenway, D., Killen, A., Cashman, S. B., Parks, C. L., & Bicknell, W. J. (1990). Physicians' responses to financial incentives: Evidence from a for-profit ambulatory care center. *The New England Journal of Medicine, 322*(15), 1059–1062.

Hetherington, R. W., Hopkins, C. E., & Roemer, M. I. (1975). *Health insurance plans: Promise and performance*. New York: Wiley-Interscience.

Heymann, J. (1995). *Equal partners*. Boston: Little, Brown.

Hillman, A. L. (1987). Financial incentives for physicians in HMOs: Is there a conflict of interest? *The New England Journal of Medicine, 317*(27), 1743–1748.

Hillman, A. L., Pauly, M. V., Kerman, K., & Martinek, C. R. (1991). HMO managers' views on financial incentives and quality. *Health Affairs, 10*(4), 207–219.

Hirsh, S. K., & Kummerow, J. (1990). *Introduction to type in organizations* (2nd ed.). Palo Alto, CA: Consulting Psychologists Press.

Holland, J. L. (1973). *Making vocational choices*. Englewood Cliffs, NJ: Prentice-Hall.

Hurdle, S., & Pope, G. C. (1989a). Improving Physician Productivity. *Journal of Ambulatory Care Management, 12*(1), 11–26.

Hurdle, S., & Pope, G. C. (1989b). Physician productivity: Trends and determinants, *Inquiry, 26*, 100–115.

Jacobson, S. (1993, May 30). California may provide answers in nation's crisis over health care; Clinton considering managed competition. *The Dallas Morning News*, p. 1A.

Jensen, J., & Larson, S. (1987). Physicians say quality of care at hospitals depends on the quality of doctors—Survey. *Modern Healthcare, 17*(11), 64–66.

Jonsen, A. (1990). *The new medicine and the old ethics*. Cambridge, MA: Harvard University Press.

Katz, P. M. (1993). Summa health plan: Why HMOs fail. In P. Boland (Ed.), *Making managed care work: A practical guide to strategies and solutions* (pp. 261–263). Gaithersburg, MD: Aspen.

Kindig, D. A., & Lastiri-Quiros, S. (1989). The changing managerial role of physician executives. *The Journal of Health Administration Education, 7*(1), 33–46.

Koch, A. L. (1993). Financing health services. In S. J. Williams & P. R. Torrens (Eds.), *Introduction to health services* (pp. 299–331). 4th ed. Albany, NY: Delmar.

Kralewski, J. E. (1995, June). Some preliminary observations regarding the impact of managed care and provider consolidation on the Minneapolis/St. Paul, Minnesota health care system. Paper presented at annual meeting of the Association for Health Services Research, Chicago, IL.

Krantz, J. (1984). The organization of professional education: A study of physician training. Doctoral dissertation, Wharton School, University of Pennsylvania, Philadelphia.

Kurtz, M. (1993). The dual role dilemma. In D. A. Kindig & A. R. Kovner (Eds.), *The role of the physician executive: Cases and commentary* (pp. 11–20). Ann Arbor, MI: Health Administration Press.

Kurtz, M. (1994). The dual role dilemma. In R. Schenke (Ed.), *New leadership in health care management* (2nd ed., pp. 81–88). Tampa, FL: The American College of Physician Executives.

Lammert, M. (1978). Power, authority, and status in health systems: A Marxian-based conflict analysis. *Journal of Applied Behavioral Science, 14*(3), 321–333.

Levit, K. R., Sensenig, A. L., Cowan, C. A., Lazenby, H. C., McDonnell, P. A., Won, D. K., Sivarajan, L., Stiller, J. M., Donham, C. S., and Stewart, M. S. (1994). National health expenditures, 1993. *Health Care Financing Review, 16*(1), 247–294.

Lewis, C. E., Prout, D. M., Chalmers, E. P., & Leake, B. (1991). How satisfying is the practice of internal medicine: A national survey. *Annals of Internal Medicine, 114*(1), 1–5.

Lewis, D. E. (1995, June 20). Surprise! You're Uninsured. *Boston Globe,* pp. 39, 58.

Lichtenstein, R. (1984). Measuring the job satisfaction of physicians in organized settings. *Medical Care, 22*(1), 56–68.

Linn, L., Brook, R., Clark, V., Davies, A., Fink, A., Kosecoff, J., & Salisbury, P. (1986). Work satisfaction and career aspirations of internists working in teaching hospital group practices. *Journal of General Internal Medicine, 1*(2), 104–108.

Lohr, K. N., Yordy, K. D., & Thier, S. O. (1988). Current issues in quality of care. *Health Affairs, 7*(1), 5–18.

Lomas, J., Anderson, G. M., Dominick-Pierre, K., Vayda, E., Enkin, M. W., & Hannah, W. J. (1989). Do practice guidelines guide practice? *The New England Journal of Medicine, 321*(19), 1306–1311.

Long, L. (1990). Americans on the move. *American Demographics, 12,* 47–49.

Luft, H. S. (1985). HMOs: Friends or foes? *Business and Health,* pp. 5–9.

Luft, H. S. (1987). *Health maintenance organizations. Dimensions of performance.* New York: Wiley.

Madison, D. L., & Konrad, T. R. (1988). Large medical group-practice organizations and employed physicians: A relationship in transition. *Milbank Quarterly/ Health and Society, 66*(2), 240–282.

Marion Merrell Dow. (1993). *Managed care digest: HMO edition, 1993.* Kansas City, MO: Marion Merrell Dow.

Marion Merrell Dow. (1994). *Managed care digest: HMO edition, 1994.* Kansas City, MO: Marion Merrell Dow.

Martin, A. R., Wolf, M. A., Thibodeau, L. A., Dzau, V., & Braunwald, E. (1980). A trial of two strategies to modify the test-ordering behavior of medical residents. *New England Journal of Medicine, 1980, 303*(23), 1330–1336.

McCarthy, E. G., & Finkel, M. (1978). Second opinion elective surgery programs: Outcome status over time. *Medical Care, 16*(12), 984–994.

McCollom, M. (1993). Comparing organizational cultures as complex wholes: A framework. *Journal of Management Inquiry, 2*(1), 83–100.

McDermott, W. (1974). General medical care: Identification and analysis of alternative approaches. *The Johns Hopkins Medical Journal, 135*(5), 292–321.

McElrath, D. C. (1961). Perspective and participation in prepaid group practice. *American Sociological Review, 26,* 596–607.

Mechanic, D. (1978). Practitioner and patient. In D. C. McElrath, *Medical Sociology* (2nd ed.). New York: Free Press, 407–432.

Menzies, I. (1975). A case-study in the functioning of social systems as a defense against anxiety. In A. Colman & H. Bexton (Eds.), *Group relations reader.* Sausalito, CA: GREX.

Merrill, M., & Moosbruker, J. (1982). Building an organizational development effort in a teaching hospital. In N. Margulies and J. Adams (Eds.), *Organizational development in health care organizations* (pp. 75–104). Reading, MA: Addison-Wesley.

Miller, E., & Rice, A. K. (1967). *Systems of organization: The control of task and sentient boundaries.* London: Tavistock Clinic.

Miller, R., & Luft, H. (1993). Managed care: Past evidence and potential trends. *Frontiers of Health Services Management, 9*(3), 3–37.

Mohrman, A., Mohrman, S. A., Ledford, G. E., Jr., Cummings, T. G., Lawler, E. E. III, & Associates (1989). *Large-scale organizational change.* San Francisco: Jossey-Bass.

More doctors look to posts with salaries, report says. (1986, December 27). *The New York Times,* p. 46.

Morgan, G. (1986). *Images of organization.* Newbury Park, CA: Sage.

Munson, F. C., & Zuckerman, H. S. (1983). The managerial role. In S. M. Shortell & A. D. Kaluzny (Eds.), *Health care management: A text in organization theory and behavior* (pp. 38–71). New York: Wiley.

Murray, J. (1988). Physician satisfaction with capitation patients in an academic family medicine clinic. *Journal of Family Practice, 27*(1), 108–113.

Nadler, D., & Tichy, N. (1982). The limitations of traditional interventional techniques in health care organizations. In N. Margulies & J. Adams (Eds.), *Organizational development in health care organizations* (pp. 359–378). Reading, MA: Addison-Wesley.

Payne, S.M.C., Ash, A., & Restuccia, J. D. (1991). The role of feedback in reducing medically unnecessary hospital use. *Medical Care, 29*(8), AS91–AS106.

Physician Payment Review Commission. (1990). *Annual report.* Washington, DC: Physician Payment Review Commission.

Plovnik, T. (1982). Structural intervention for health systems' organizational development. In N. Margulies & J. Adams (Eds.), *Organizational development in health care organizations*. Reading, MA: Addison-Wesley.

Pope, G. C., & Schneider, J. E. (1992). Trends in physician income. *Health Affairs, 11*(1), 181–193.

Porter, L., & Lawler, E. E. (1965). Properties of organization structure in relation to job attitudes and behavior. *Psychological Bulletin*, pp. 23–51.

Porter L., & Steers, R. (1973). Organizational, work and personal factors in employee turnover and absenteeism. *Psychological Bulletin, 80*(2), 151–176.

Prybil, L. (1971). Physician terminations in large multispecialty groups. *Medical Group Management, 18*(5,6).

Raelin, J. A. (1985). *The clash of cultures*. Boston: Harvard Business School Press.

Reames, H. R., & Dunstone, D. C. (1989). Professional satisfaction of physicians. *Archives of Internal Medicine, 149*, 1951–1956.

Relman, A. (1992). Self-referral: What's at stake? *New England Journal of Medicine, 327*(21), 1522–1523.

Restuccia, J. D. (1982). The effect of concurrent feedback in reducing inappropriate hospital utilization. *Medical Care, 20*(1), 46–62.

Restuccia, J. D., & Holloway, D. C. (1982). Methods of control for hospital quality assurance systems. *Health Services Research, 17*(3), 241–268.

Richardsen, A., & Burke. R. (1991). Occupational stress and job satisfaction among physicians. *Social Science and Medicine, 33*(10), 1179–1187.

Roback, E., Randolph, L., & Seidman, B. (1993). *Physician characteristics and distribution in the U.S.* Chicago: American Medical Association.

Rodwin, M. (1993). *Medicine, money and morals: Physicians' conflicts of interest*. New York: Oxford University Press.

Roemer, M. I., & Shonick, W. (1973). HMO performance: The recent evidence. *Milbank Quarterly, 51*(3), 271–317.

Rogers, C., & Farson, R. (1976). *Active listening.* Chicago: Industrial Relations Center of the University of Chicago.

Rohrer, J. E. (1989). The secret of medical management. *Health Care Management Review, 14*(3), 7–13.

Rose, C. (1993, April 11). Interview, CNN.

Rosenfeld, S. C. (1994, August 9). So you want to join an HMO? Good luck. *The New York Times,* p. A23.

Ross, A. (1969). A report on physician terminations in group practice. *Medical Group Management, 16*(5), 15–21.

Rothman, D. J. (1991). *Strangers at the bedside: A history of how law and bioethics transformed medical decisionmaking.* New York: Basic Books.

Rothman, D. J. (1993). Who's in charge here? *Health Management Quarterly,* pp. 17–21.

Russell, S. (1995, February 21). Consumers feel sting of newest HMO cost cuts: Hundreds of specialists dropped from the rolls. *San Francisco Chronicle,* p. 1.

Satow, R. (1975). Value-rational authority and professional organizations: Weber's missing type. *Administrative Science Quarterly, 20*(4), 526–531.

Schön, D. (1983). *The reflective practitioner.* New York: Basic Books.

Schroeder, S. A. (1992). Physician supply and the U.S. medical marketplace. *Health Affairs, 11*(1), 235–243.

Schulz, R., Girard, C., & Scheckler, W. E. (1992). Physician satisfaction in a managed care environment. *Journal of Family Practice, 3,* 298–304.

Schulz, R., Grimes, D. S., & Chester, T. E. (1976). Physician participation in health service management: Expectations in United States and experiences in England. *Milbank Quarterly/Health and Society, 55,* 107–127.

Scott, W. R. (1966). Some implications of organization theory for research on health services. *Milbank Quarterly, 44*(4), 35–59.

Scott, W. R. (1982). Managing professional work: Three models of control for health organizations. *Health Services Research, 17*(3), 213–240.

Senge, P. (1990). *The fifth discipline.* New York: Doubleday.

Sherer, J. L. (1993). Physician CEOs: Ranks continue to grow. *Hospitals, 67*(9), 42.

Shortell, S. M., & Kaluzny, A. D. (1983). Organizational theory and health care management. In S. M. Shortell & A. D. Kaluzny (Eds.), *Health care management: A text in organization theory and behavior* (pp. 5–37). New York: Wiley.

Shortell, S. M., O'Brien, J. L., Carman, J. M., Foster, R. W., Hughes, E.F.X., Boerstler, H., O'Connor, E. J., & Gillies, R. R. (1995). Physician involvement in quality improvement: Issues, challenges, and recommendations. In D. Blumenthal & A. C. Scheck (Eds.), *Improving clinical practice: Total quality management and the physician* (pp. 205–228). San Francisco: Jossey-Bass.

Smith, H. L., Reid, R. A., & Piland, N. F. (1990). Managing hospital-physician relations: A strategy scorecard. *Health Care Management Review, 15*(4), 23–33.

Society for Human Resource Management. (1990). *Health care cost containment survey.*

Steptoe, S. (1987, April 10). Dispirited doctors: Hassles and red tape destroy joy of the job for many physicians. *The Wall Street Journal,* p. A1.

Stevens, F., Diederiks, J., & Philipsen, H. (1992). Physician satisfaction, professional characteristics, and behavior formalization in hospitals. *Social Science and Medicine, 35*(3), 295–303.

Stoeckle, J. D., & Reiser, S. J. (1992). The corporate organization of hospital work: balancing professional and administrative responsibilities. *Annals of Internal Medicine, 116*(5), 407–413.

Stoelwinder, J. (1982, June). Hospital management—What's the point? Paper presented to the 9th annual congress, Australian College of Health Service Administrators.

Stoelwinder, J., & Clayton, P. (1978). Hospital organization development: Changing the focus from "better management" to "better patient care." *Journal of Applied Behavioral Science, 14*(3), 400–413.

Sullivan, C. B., Miller, M., Feldman, R., & Dowd, B. (1992). Employer-sponsored health insurance in 1991. *Health Affairs, 11*(4), 172–185.

Sutherland, V., & Cooper, C. (1993). Identifying distress among general practitioners: Predictors of psychological ill-health and job dissatisfaction. *Social Science and Medicine, 37*(5), 575–581.

Swedlow, A., Johnson, G., Smithline, N., & Milstein, A. (1992). Increased costs and rates of use in the California workers' compensation system as a result of self-referral by physicians. *New England Journal of Medicine, 327*(21), 1502–1506.

Tabenkin, H., Zyzanski, S. J., & Alemagno, S. A. (1989). Physician managers: Personal characteristics versus institutional demands. *Health Care Management Review, 14*(2), 7–12.

Tieger, P., & Barron-Tieger, B. (1992). *Do what you are.* Boston: Little, Brown.

Tucker, C. J., & Urton, W. (1987). Frequency of geographic mobility: Findings from the national health interview survey. *Demography, 24*(2), 265–270.

U.S. Bureau of the Census. (1994). *Statistical abstract of the United States, 1994.* Washington, DC: U.S. Department of Commerce.

Veatch, R. M. (1977). *Case studies in medical ethics.* Cambridge, MA: Harvard University Press.

Von Bertalanffy, L. (1968). General systems theory: Foundations, development, applications. New York: Braziller.

Wallace, C. (1987). Physicians leaving their practices for hospital jobs. *Modern Healthcare, 17*(10), 40–57.

Weisbord, M. (1976). Why organizational development hasn't worked (so far) in medical centers. *Health Care Management Review, 1*(2), 17–38.

Weisbord, M., & Goodstein, L. (1978). Introduction: Towards healthier medical systems: Can we learn from experience? *Journal of Applied Behavioral Science*, *14*(3), 263–264.

Weisbord, M., Lawrence, P., & Charns, M. (1978). Three dilemmas of academic medical centers. *Journal of Applied Behavioral Science*, *14*(3), 284–304.

Welch, W. P., Hillman, A. L., & Pauly, M. V. (1990). Toward new typologies for HMOs. *The Milbank Quarterly*, *68*(2), 221–243.

Wenzel, R. P. (1994, March 27). Health plan must preserve doctor-patient ties. *The New York Times*, News of the Week Section, p. 16.

Wheelwright, S. C. (1984). Manufacturing strategy: Defining the missing link. *Strategic Management Journal*, *5*, 77–91.

Wilensky, G. R., & Rossiter, L. F. (1983). The relative importance of physician-induced demand in the demand for medical care. *Milbank Quarterly*, *2*, 252–277.

Willke, R. J., & Cotter, P. S. (1989). Young physicians and changes in medical practice characteristics between 1975 and 1987. *Inquiry*, *26*(1), 84–99.

Wirth, T., & Allcorn, S. (1993). *Creating new hospital-physician collaboration*. Ann Arbor, MI: Health Administration Press.

Wolfe, D., & Kolb, D. (1984). Career development, personal growth, and experiential learning. In D. Kolb, I. Rubin, & J. McIntyre (Eds.), *Organizational psychology* (pp. 124–152.). 4th ed. Englewood Cliffs, NJ: Prentice-Hall.

# Index